JN299529

Drug-Induced Suffering in Japan

A Review from Regulatory and Social Perspectives

日本の薬害事件

薬事規制と社会的要因からの考察

企画・編集　一般財団法人 医薬品医療機器レギュラトリーサイエンス財団

Edited by Pharmaceutical and Medical Device Regulatory Science Society of Japan

薬事日報社
YAKUJI NIPPO, LTD.

はじめに

　本書は，第二次世界大戦後の日本における主な薬害事件を取り上げたものです。その狙いは一連の事件を俯瞰することによって，歴史から何ものかを学ぶことにあります。これまで個々の薬害事例については，多くの研究書や啓発書がありますので詳細はそちらに譲りますが，薬害史を俯瞰しようという試みは多くはありません。私たちは2010年，「日本における医薬品のリスクマネジメント」という対訳本を出版しました。その本では日本の薬事制度の変遷と要点を主眼として扱いました。そして本書はその姉妹本になります。

　中国の孔子の言葉に「温故而知新,可以為師矣」というものがあります。英語では「Those who review what they have learnt will know something new, and they can be teachers.」と訳されています。一方，ドイツのビスマルクの言葉に「愚者は経験に学び，賢者は歴史に学ぶ(Nur ein Idiot glaubt, aus den eigenen Erfahrungen zu lernen. Ich ziehe es vor, aus den Erfahrungen anderer zu lernen, um von vorneherein eigene Fehler zu vermeiden.)」というものがあります。英語ではFools say they learn from experience; I prefer to learn from the experience of others.と訳されています。この二つの言葉の間には2500年以上の隔たりがあるにも関わらず，私たちは自分の経験だけに頼るのではなく，空間的にも時間的にも広く事象を訪ねて学ばなくてはならない，という真理を表しています。

　本書を企画した一つの動機は，日本で発生した肝炎薬害事件を検証した提言でした。2010年に公表されたこの提言では，薬害教育が医学・薬学生はもとより医療関係者，製薬企業の経営者を含む全従業員になされるべきであると指摘しています。しかし，残念ながら日本においてこの提言の趣旨に沿う，薬害教育に関する適切なテキストがありませんでした。そこで私たちの財団では日本の薬害事件を10巻のDVDとして編集，出版するプロジェクトを2012年より開始し，これまでに4巻を出版しました。

　もう一つの動機は，薬害事件というものは日本以外の国々でも発生していながらその多くを知らないと同様に，日本の薬害事件については断片的にしか海外に伝えられていないのではないかということでした。日本では多くの薬害事件が，国と製薬企業を被告とする裁判へと発展しています。その教訓を活かして，政府はその都度，薬事制度の改善を行い，現在の開発，審査から市販後までの一貫したライフサイクルリスクマネジメントの制度を確立してきました。医学，薬学はサイエンスとして世界の共通語であり認識でありま

PREFACE

This book focuses on major incidents of damage to health caused by drugs or medical devices that have occurred in Japan since the end of World War II. The aim is to provide a bird's eye overview of these incidents from both regulatory and social perspectives so as to learn lessons from this unfortunate history. Although many research articles and enlightening books on the individual incidents have already documented much of the detail, which the reader may want to refer to for the details, only a few of them have tried to make a comprehensive overview of the history of drug-induced suffering in Japan. In 2010, we published a book entitled "Drug Risk Management in Japan" written in Japanese with an accompanying English translation. The 2010 book is primarily concerned with changes and essential points of the Japanese pharmaceutical regulatory system. This is its sister book.

One of the teachings by the Chinese philosopher, Confucius (Kong Zi), is "wen gu er zhi xin ke yi wei shi yi", which translates into English as: "Those who review what they have learnt will know something new, and they can be teachers". The first chancellor of the united German Empire, Otto von Bismarck, said that "Nur ein Idiot glaubt, aus den eigenen Erfahrungen zu lernen. Ich ziehe es vor, aus den Erfahrungen anderer zu lernen, um von voneherein eigene Fehler zu vermeiden", which translates as: "Fools say they learn from experience; I prefer to learn from the experience of others". These two sayings, which originate over 2,500 years apart, represent the truth that we should not depend on our own experience alone but seek and learn from others, drawing on lessons over a wide range of events that take place at different places and time.

What made us plan this book was the official proposal announced by the special committee that had verified the drug-induced hepatitis events in Japan. The proposal was made public in 2010 and pointed out the necessity of providing education about drug-induced suffering to not only students at medical and pharmaceutical schools but also healthcare professionals and all employees of pharmaceutical companies including the management. Unfortunately, in Japan, there were no adequate textbooks meeting the intention of this proposal regarding the education. We, the Pharmaceutical and Medical Device Regulatory Science Society of Japan, started a project of editing and publishing a set of 10 DVDs which outline incidents of drug-induced suffering in Japan. The project was started in 2012 and we have released 4 DVDs so far.

In addition, we consider that drug-induced sufferings have occurred also in many foreign countries, and in Japan there is a lack of awareness of such overseas incidents, and vice versa. Only fragmentary information on the incidents of drug-induced health damage in Japan is made known

すが医療は文化であり，今なお地域性を強く持ったものです。そして薬害事件は医療文化の負の部分であるがゆえに，国境を越えた共通認識になりにくいのであろうと思います。私たちは日本の経験を海外に発信し共有する責任があると考えました。

　私たちはこの二つの動機から企画した本書が先に出版した姉妹本と併せて，海外の行政当局，企業，医療関係者に読まれ，医薬品や医療機器によるリスクを低減するための公共政策に少しでも参考となることを願っています。

(一財)医薬品医療機器レギュラトリーサイエンス財団
理事長　土井　脩

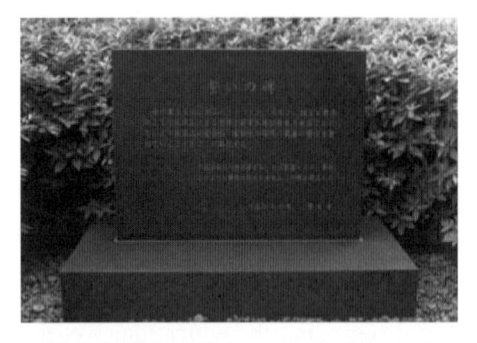

誓いの碑

　命の尊さを心に刻みサリドマイド，スモン，HIV感染のような医薬品による悲惨な被害を再び発生させることのないよう医薬品の安全性・有効性の確保に最善の努力を重ねていくことをここに銘記する

厚生労働省敷地内に建てられた「薬害根絶のための『誓いの碑』」です。1999年8月24日に完成し，除幕されました。

overseas. In Japan, many of the drug-induced sufferings brought about lawsuits in which the defendants included the national government and pharmaceutical companies. By making the best use of the lessons from these lawsuits, the Japanese government revised its pharmaceutical regulatory system as appropriate, and has formulated a currently effective life-cycle risk management system covering the whole process from development, review and approval, through to post-marketing. On the other hand, medicine and pharmacology functions as a common language and understanding as science all over the world, whereas healthcare represents culture and greatly depends on regions still at present. Drug-induced sufferings form a negative aspect of healthcare culture and that is why these incidents are unlikely to become a shared understanding between different countries. We should inform people outside Japan of what Japanese have experienced so as to share our experience with people overseas. This is the second motive for planning this book.

We genuinely hope that this book, born from the above two motives, together with the previously published sister book, is read by overseas administrative agencies, companies, and healthcare professionals, and provides useful information to them when they formulate their own public policies to reduce the risks related to drugs and medical devices.

Chief Executive Osamu Doi Ph.D.
Pharmaceutical and Medical Device Regulatory Science Society of Japan (PMRJ)

〔Epigraph〕
Taking preciousness of life at heart, we hereby declare that we will make our best effort to secure the safety and efficacy of drugs to prevent recurrence of thalidomide, SMON disease, HIV infection, and other tragic incidents of suffering caused by drugs.

〔Explanation of the photo〕
This is the "Monument of Oath for Eradication of Drug-Induced Suffering" unveiled in the premises of the Ministry of Health, Labour and Welfare on August 24, 1999.

目　次

- 第1章　薬害の定義の試み 1
- 第2章　日本の薬害事件 9
  1. ジフテリア予防接種禍事件 10
  2. ペニシリンショック事件 14
  3. サリドマイド事件 18
  4. アンプル入り風邪薬事件 24
  5. スモン事件 30
  6. 筋短縮症事件 38
  7. ダイアライザーによる眼障害事件 44
  8. エイズ事件 48
  9. 血液製剤（フィブリノゲン製剤）によるHCV感染事件 56
  10. 陣痛促進剤事件 64
  11. MMRワクチン事件 70
  12. ソリブジン事件 76
  13. ヒト乾燥硬膜によるプリオン感染（CJD）事件 84
  14. ウシ心嚢膜抗酸菌様感染事件 88
  15. ゲフィチニブ事件 92
- 第3章　日本の薬害事件の概括と分析 103
- 第4章　参考資料 135
  1. 薬害再発防止のための医薬品行政の見直しについての概要 136
  2. 緊急安全性情報（イエローレター）と発出の実績 152
  3. 医薬品リスク管理計画指針について 156
  4. 医薬品リスク管理計画の策定について 180
  5. 薬害に関する公的教育について 224
  6. 全国薬害被害者団体連絡協議会 228
  7. 承認条件 232
  8. 市販直後調査制度 240
  9. 医薬品副作用被害救済制度の概要 242
  10. PMDAの理念 246
  11. 日本の薬害年表 248

Contents

Chapter 1   DEFINING "DRUG-INDUCED SUFFERING (YAKUGAI)" ················ 1

Chapter 2   DRUG-INDUCED SUFFERING IN JAPAN ································ 9
    1. Diphtheria Immunization Incident ·· 11
    2. Penicillin Shock Incident ·· 15
    3. Thalidomide Incident ··· 19
    4. Cold-Medicines-in-Ampoules Incident ······································ 25
    5. SMON Incident ·· 31
    6. Muscle Contracture Incident ·· 39
    7. Dialyzer Induced Ophthalmologic Disorders Incident ··················· 45
    8. AIDS Incident ·· 49
    9. Blood Product (Fibrinogen) Induced HCV Infection Incident ········· 57
    10. Labor-Inducing Drugs Incident ··· 65
    11. MMR Vaccine Incident ··· 71
    12. Sorivudine Incident ··· 77
    13. Human Dried Dura Mater Induced Prion Infection (CJD) Incident ······· 85
    14. Incident of Bovine Pericardium Induced Infection with Probably Acid-Fast Bacilli ········ 89
    15. Gefitinib Incident ··· 93

Chapter 3   OVERVIEW AND ANALYSIS OF DRUG-INDUCED SUFFERING IN JAPAN ································ 103

Chapter 4   REFERENCE DATA ································ 135
    1. Summary of the Review of the Drug Administration for Preventing Recurrence of Drug-induced Sufferings ········· 137
    2. Previously Issued Urgent Safety Information (Yellow Letter) ········ 153
    3. Risk Management Plan Guidance ·· 157
    4. Development of Risk Management Plan ·································· 181
    5. Public Education of Drug-Induced Suffering ····························· 225
    6. Japanese National Liaison Council for Associations of Victims of Drug-Induced Suffering ··············· 229
    7. Conditional Approval System ·· 233
    8. Early Post-marketing Phase Risk Minimization and Vigilance (EPRV) system ········ 241
    9. Summary of the Relief Service for Adverse Drug Reactions ········ 243
    10. Our philosophy (PMDA) ·· 247
    11. Chronological Table of Drug-Induced Suffering in Japan ············· 249

〈関係組織の沿革〉

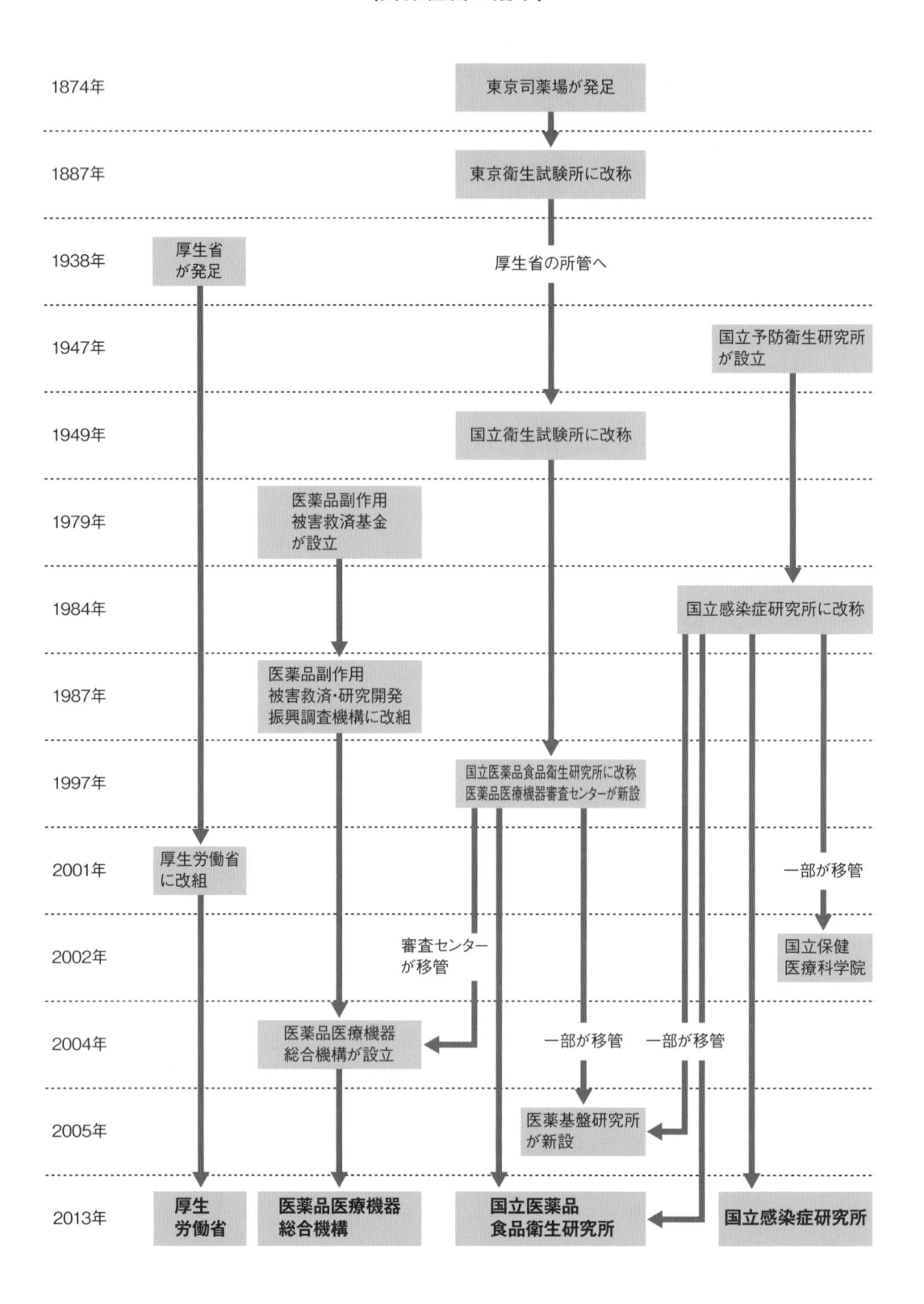

1874年	東京司薬場が発足
1887年	東京衛生試験所に改称
1938年	厚生省が発足 → 厚生省の所管へ
1947年	国立予防衛生研究所が設立
1949年	国立衛生試験所に改称
1979年	医薬品副作用被害救済基金が設立
1984年	国立感染症研究所に改称
1987年	医薬品副作用被害救済・研究開発振興調査機構に改組
1997年	国立医薬品食品衛生研究所に改称／医薬品医療機器審査センターが新設
2001年	厚生労働省に改組
2002年	審査センターが移管／一部が移管 → 国立保健医療科学院
2004年	医薬品医療機器総合機構が設立
2005年	医薬基盤研究所が新設（一部が移管）
2013年	厚生労働省／医薬品医療機器総合機構／国立医薬品食品衛生研究所／国立感染症研究所

⟨History of related organizations⟩

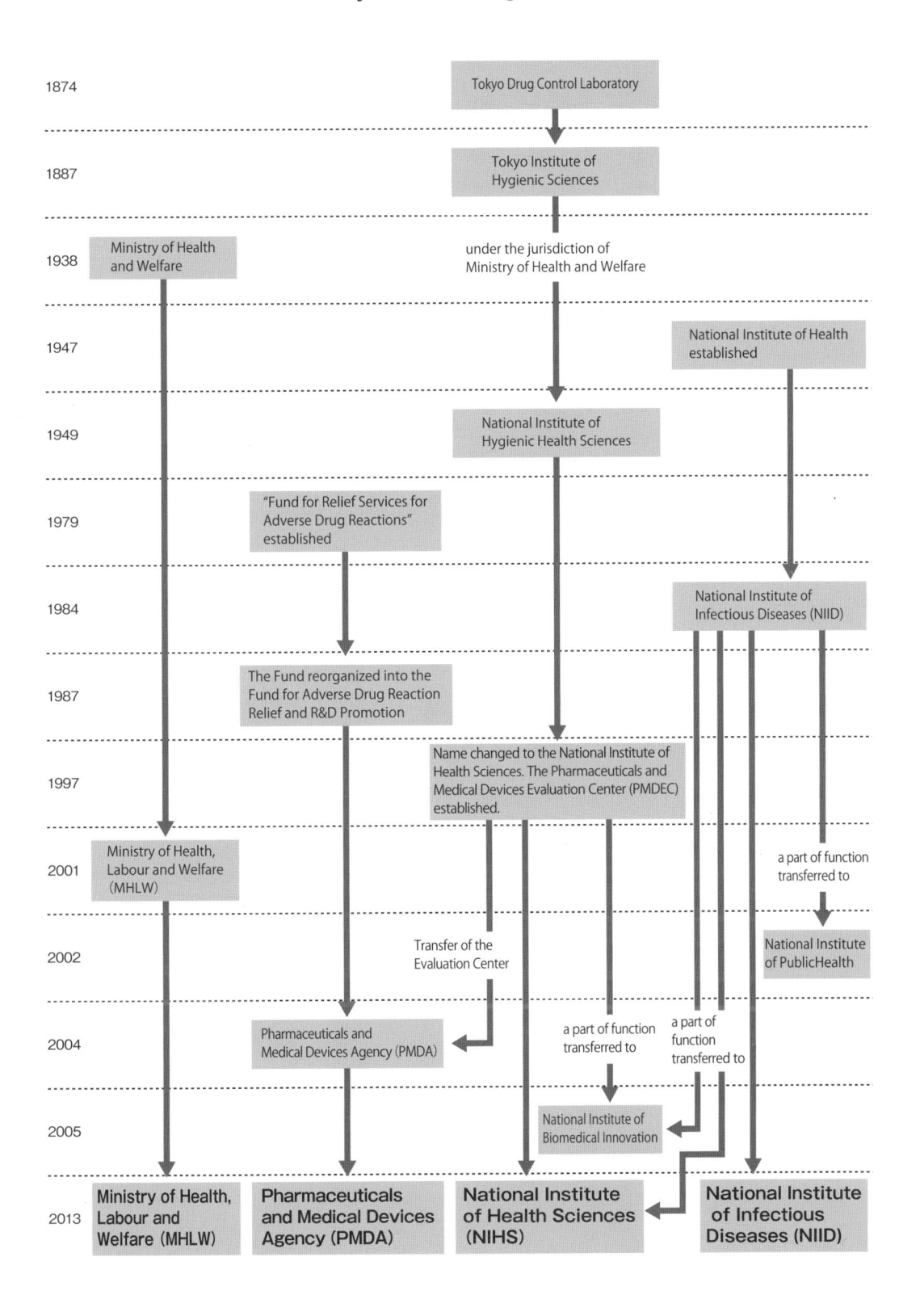

1874			Tokyo Drug Control Laboratory	
1887			Tokyo Institute of Hygienic Sciences	
1938	Ministry of Health and Welfare		under the jurisdiction of Ministry of Health and Welfare	
1947				National Institute of Health established
1949			National Institute of Hygienic Health Sciences	
1979		"Fund for Relief Services for Adverse Drug Reactions" established		
1984				National Institute of Infectious Diseases (NIID)
1987		The Fund reorganized into the Fund for Adverse Drug Reaction Relief and R&D Promotion		
1997			Name changed to the National Institute of Health Sciences. The Pharmaceuticals and Medical Devices Evaluation Center (PMDEC) established.	
2001	Ministry of Health, Labour and Welfare (MHLW)			a part of function transferred to
2002		Transfer of the Evaluation Center		National Institute of Public Health
2004		Pharmaceuticals and Medical Devices Agency (PMDA)	a part of function transferred to	a part of function transferred to
2005			National Institute of Biomedical Innovation	
2013	**Ministry of Health, Labour and Welfare (MHLW)**	**Pharmaceuticals and Medical Devices Agency (PMDA)**	**National Institute of Health Sciences (NIHS)**	**National Institute of Infectious Diseases (NIID)**

chapter 1

薬害の定義の試み

DEFINING "DRUG-INDUCED SUFFERING (YAKUGAI)"

薬害という言葉は文字通りに英訳すれば，Drug hazardとかDrug safety scandalとなるのでしょう。しかし，Scandalという言葉は興味本位に受け止められる可能性がありますので，私たちが2010年に出版した「日本における医薬品のリスクマネジメント（Drug Risk Management in Japan）」では，薬害という言葉にDrug induced sufferingという訳語をあてました。日本語で薬害（YAKUGAI）という言葉は，文字どおりにはYAKU（Drug）とGAI（Hazard）という言葉の組み合わせです。しかし単に薬による健康被害という以上に，社会的に問題になった事件というニュアンスがあります。この言葉は第二次大戦後に使われるようになりましたが，「薬害」の公式な定義は，日本にありません。以下に，私たちはその定義を試みたいと思います。

被害の規模や深刻さから，副作用による健康被害を以下の4つのカテゴリーに分類します。

〈カテゴリー1〉

医薬品は本質的に健康被害を避けられないものです。適応症，用法用量，使用上の注意を守っていても（日本では，これをせまい意味での"適正使用"としています），散発的に孤立して発生する健康被害があります。この種の健康被害をカテゴリー1としますが，薬害という概念には含まれません。この種の健康被害は，日本では健康被害救済の対象となっています（ただし，抗がん剤などリストアップされた特定の医薬品によるものを除く）。

〈カテゴリー2〉

適応症，用法用量，使用上の注意を守っていれば防げたはずの健康被害です。適正使用の指示を守らなかったので，一般には医療過誤・医療事故として捉えられます。したがって健康被害救済の対象とはならず，時に医療訴訟に発展することがあります。医薬品の使用法を改め，適正使用を徹底することにより重篤な副作用を回避し，発生時にはその健康被害を最小限度に抑え込むために添付文書改訂，緊急安全性情報の発出等が行われます。健康被害が社会問題化しなければこのカテゴリーに収まっていますが，防ぎえる健康被害という意味では，その防止対策は非常に大切です。このカテゴリーの健康被害も，通常は薬害には含まれません。

The Japanese term "YAKUGAI" can be literally translated into English as "drug hazard" or "drug safety scandal". However, since we are cautious that the term "scandal" may attract people's attention out of curiosity and not as a serious issue, we decided to use the English phrase of "drug-induced suffering" when we published the book entitled "Drug Risk Management in Japan" in 2010. The Japanese term "YAKUGAI" is a combination of "YAKU" (which means "drug") and "GAI" ("hazard"). The term "drug-induced suffering" does not only indicate health damage caused by adverse drug reactions but also implies a nuance that these incidents have become social issues. This term began to be used after the end of World War II in Japan, although there is no official definition of the term "drug-induced suffering". We therefore attempt to define it as described below.

Depending on scale and seriousness, health damage events caused by adverse drug reactions are included in one of the following four categories.

⟨Category 1⟩

Due to their nature, drugs may unavoidably cause damage to health in some instances. Even though a drug is used in strict accordance with the officially approved instructions on indication(s), dosage and administration, and precautions for use (note that in Japan, this use is referred to as "proper use" in a narrow sense), damage to health may occur in an isolated and sporadic manner. This type of health damage is defined as "Category 1" but is not included in the concept of "drug-induced suffering". In Japan, this type of health damage is covered by the relief services system for adverse health effects (although this system is not applicable to specifically listed drugs such as anticancer agents).

⟨Category 2⟩

Health damage events which should have been avoided if the officially approved instructions on indication(s), dosage and administration, and precautions for use had been followed are included in "Category 2". These events are generally regarded as medical malpractice or medical accident since the instructions on the proper use are not followed. These events are therefore not covered by the relief services system for adverse health effects and sometimes bring about lawsuits. For the purposes of correcting the use of a drug and fully disseminating the proper use of the drug so as to avoid serious adverse reactions and minimize health damage caused by adverse drug reactions if they should occur, revision of the package insert of the drug, issuance of an Urgent Safety Information regarding the drug, and any other relevant actions are taken. If a health damage event does not become a social issue, the event remains in this Category. Since health damage events in Category 2 could have been avoided, it is important to take preventive actions against such health

▶医薬品等による健康被害

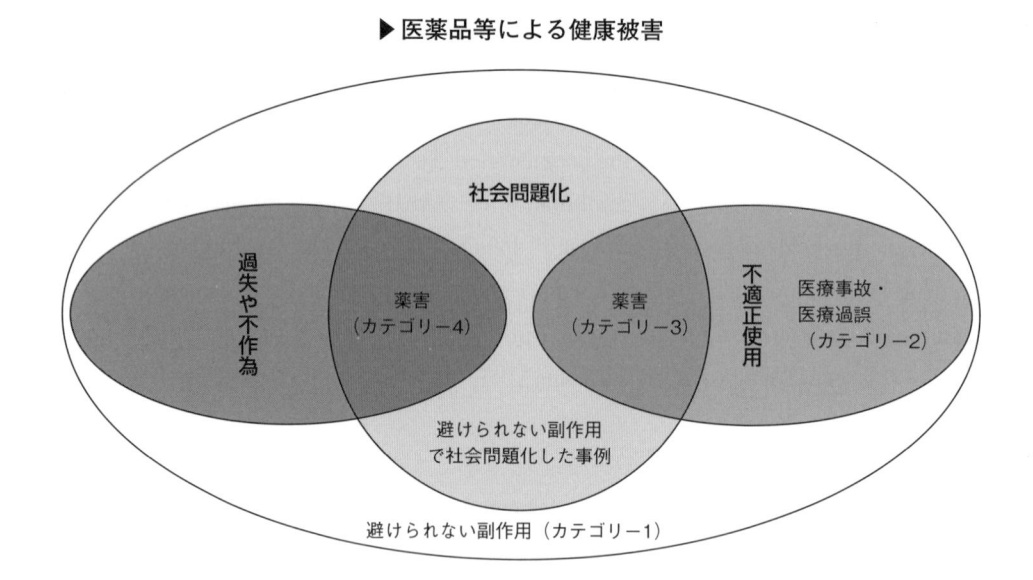

図中:
- 社会問題化
- 過失や不作為
- 薬害（カテゴリー4）
- 薬害（カテゴリー3）
- 不適正使用
- 医療事故・医療過誤（カテゴリー2）
- 避けられない副作用で社会問題化した事例
- 避けられない副作用（カテゴリー1）

〈カテゴリー3〉

　適正使用されていれば防げた健康被害（カテゴリー2）のうち，不確定な社会的要因が絡んで，被害が社会的に拡大した健康被害です。このカテゴリーの健康被害は一般に薬害に入る事例となります。カテゴリー2と3の違いは必ずしも明確ではありません。

〈カテゴリー4〉

　健康被害を加速，拡大する要因のうち，特に行政や承認を有する企業等の瑕疵，不作為が大きな要因を占めると指摘される場合には，その健康被害の規模は大きくなり，ほとんどが大規模な訴訟に発展しています。

　以上のカテゴリーに分類される典型的な薬害（カテゴリー3及び4）には，複数の社会的要因が絡んでいます。したがって，その様相は事件ごとに多様になります。そのため，薬害発生の予防や最小化について誰が最終責任を持つのか，ということについて社会的コンセンサスが不十分かもしれません。そしてそのコントロールはどこまで可能なのか，ということも試行錯誤の段階です。2013年4月から新薬の市販要件となったリスクマネジメントプラン（RMP）の提出も，新たな試行錯誤の一つといえます。

▶ Health damage caused by drugs, etc.

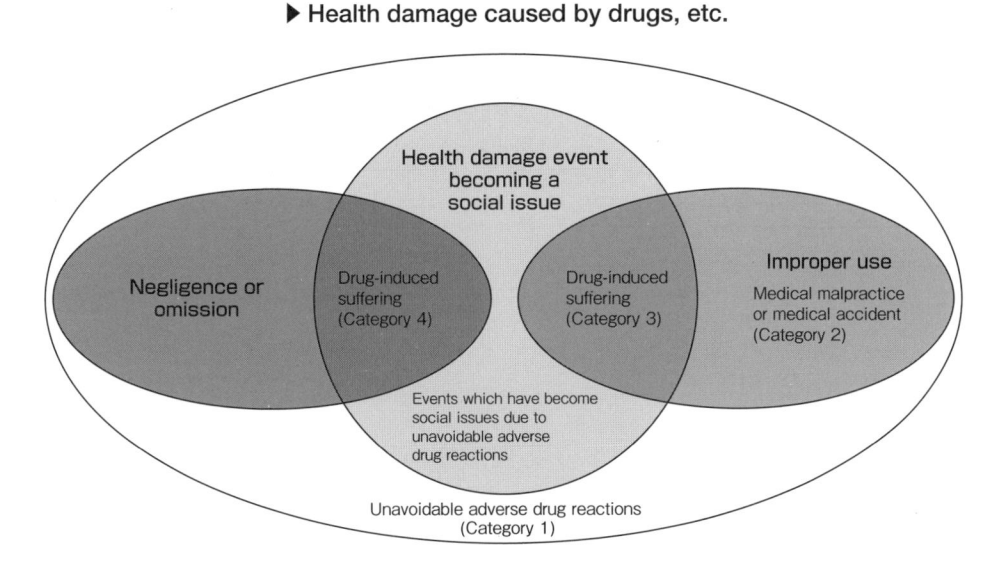

[Venn diagram showing overlapping categories of health damage:]
- Health damage event becoming a social issue
- Negligence or omission
- Drug-induced suffering (Category 4)
- Drug-induced suffering (Category 3)
- Improper use — Medical malpractice or medical accident (Category 2)
- Events which have become social issues due to unavoidable adverse drug reactions
- Unavoidable adverse drug reactions (Category 1)

damage. Generally, the damage to health in this Category is not included in the definition of drug-induced suffering.

〈Category 3〉

Among health damage events which should have been avoided if the proper use had been strictly observed (i.e. Category 2), those that cause health damage to an expanded segment of society due to involvement of uncertain social factors are included in this Category. The health damage in this Category is usually considered as drug-induced suffering. We cannot always differentiate clearly between Categories 2 and 3.

〈Category 4〉

When a fault or omission of the drug administration or marketing authorization holders accounts for a greater portion of the factors accelerating and expanding health damage caused by adverse drug reactions, the scale of such health damage increases. Almost all such health damage events develop into large-scale lawsuits.

In typical drug-induced sufferings included in Categories 3 and 4 above, multiple social factors are involved. For this reason individual incidents of drug-induced suffering are diverse in terms of their progression and the circumstances surrounding the situation. This may explain that social consensus is insufficient regarding the issue of who should take final responsibility for preventing and minimizing the onset of drug-induced suffering. To what extent we can control the prevention and minimization is now in the stage of trial and error. The Risk Management Plan (RMP) that an

第2章では戦後の日本で発生した薬害の個々の事例を取り上げます。そしてその薬害をきっかけとして日本の薬事制度が変遷，発展してきた状況について言及します。第3章では取り上げた薬害事例の全体を俯瞰して，共通する要素，要因はなにか，ということを考察していきます。

applicant for marketing authorization for a new drug shall submit to the regulatory authorities when submitting the approval application in or after April 2013 also represents a new form of trial and error.

Chapter 2 summarizes individual incidents of drug-induced suffering that have occurred in Japan since the end of World War II, and describes how the Japanese pharmaceutical regulatory system has changed and developed due to these incidents. Chapter 3 takes a 'bird's-eye' overview of these incidents and discusses the common elements or factors to them.

chapter 2

日本の薬害事件

DRUG-INDUCED SUFFERING IN JAPAN

　第2章では戦後日本で発生した15の薬害事件を取り上げます。これらは健康被害の内容，規模，原因と目される要素等は様々です。読者の時間的な理解を助けるために，第4章に事件の発生等を年表の形にまとめました。薬害は社会的に発見（認知）されるまでに，既に拡大していることもありますが，その正確な時期を特定するのは困難です。年表には社会的に認知された年から裁判で決着するなど，マイルストーンがはっきりしている時期までをその薬害の期間としました。

In Chapter 2, 15 incidents of damage to health caused by drugs or medical devices that have occurred in Japan since the end of World War II are summarized. Each incident is different in terms of history, scale, probable causes, and other relevant factors behind the health damage. A chronological table of these incidents and other prominent events is provided at the end of Chapter 4 for the purpose of helping the reader better understand the context of the incidents over time. It is difficult to exactly determine duration of drug-induced suffering since it may have already expanded substantially when eventually discovered or acknowledged by society. The durations of incidents shown in this table are therefore based on milestones, e.g. a period between a particular year in which an incident was recognized by society and the time at which a court made its decision in a lawsuit.

1 ジフテリア予防接種禍事件

事件の概要

　1945年8月，日本はポツダム宣言を受諾して第二次世界大戦は終了しました。その当時の日本は戦争により社会は疲弊し，栄養状態や衛生状態は極めて悪い状態でした。当時，日本にはジフテリアが蔓延していました。1946年2月，当時の日本を占領していたGHQ（連合国最高司令官総司令部）は，日本における感染症対策の一つとして「ジフテリア予防接種に関する覚書」を発表しました。これを受けて，1948年には予防接種法が制定されました。この法律は3,000円の罰金つき義務接種という，世界でも例のない強制力をもった予防接種法でした（当時の国家公務員の月給は13,000円）。

　事件は1948年10月と11月，全国で最初にジフテリアの予防接種が行われた京都府で発生しました。京都では10万人の乳幼児に接種され，606人が発症，うち68人が死亡しました。生存した被害者のうち538人に後遺症が残りました。この京都の事件の後に引き続いて島根県で接種が行われましたが，同様に248人が発症し，16人が死亡しました。京都府と島根県の健康被害を合わせると被害者854人，うち死亡者84人という世界最大規模の予防接種事故とされています。

　この予防接種には日本で製造されたジフテリアトキソイドが使われましたが，ホルマリンによる無毒化が十分でないロットが含まれていました。しかも，問題のあるロットを国家検定で発見できなかったのです。当時の製造記録から国家検定に合格しないロットがたびたび製造されており，当時の製造技術，品質管理が十分でなかったことがうかがわれます。問題のあるロットが国家検定をすり抜けた原因は今もはっきりしていませんが，規定に従ったランダムサンプリングができていれば，問題のあるロットを見逃す可能性は確率的にほとんどありえないことが検証されています。

　京都府の事件発生から島根県での事件発生までに，時間的間隔はほとんどありません。当時の厚生省と島根県は京都の事件を受けて問題のあるロットを疑い，それ以外のロットであれば安全と判断して，島根県で予防接種を継続しました。しかし，実際には国家検定がずさんであったために，安全だと判断したロットも不良品だったのです。

　この事件は裁判となりましたが，他の薬害裁判と大きく異なる点があります。不良品を

1 Diphtheria Immunization Incident

Summary of the incident

In August 1945, Japan accepted the Potsdam Declaration and surrendered to the Allies, bringing an end to World War II. In those days, the Japanese society was exhausted by the war effort and the people were in extremely bad conditions in terms of nutrition and hygiene. Diphtheria was sweeping Japan. In February 1946, the General Headquarters, Supreme Commander for the Allied Powers (GHQ/SCAP), the agency of occupation in Japan, issued the "Memorandum on Diphtheria Immunization" as a measure to control infection in Japan, leading to the enactment of the Preventive Vaccination Law in 1948. This law was unique in the world because of its forced vaccination; the law made it mandatory to undergo vaccination and anyone who did not receive a vaccine was liable to a fine of three thousand Japanese Yen (3,000 Yen)(compared to a monthly salary of 13,000 Japanese Yen for a national public official at that time).

In October and November 1948, the diphtheria immunization incident occurred in Kyoto Prefecture where the diphtheria immunization was performed first all over Japan. Of 100,000 infants and children given the inoculation in Kyoto, 606 experienced reactions of varying degrees of severity and 68 of them died. Of the survivors, 538 suffered from sequelae. Following the incident in Kyoto, the immunization was conducted in Shimane Prefecture, resulting in 248 sufferers and 16 deaths. Combined, Kyoto and Shimane totaled 854 sufferers, of whom 84 died. This is the world's largest such scale of incident due to immunization.

This immunization used diphtheria toxoid manufactured in Japan. Some lots of the toxoid were incompletely detoxified with formalin and this toxic material was distributed for inoculation since the national inspection failed to identify the problem. The manufacturing records at that time revealed that lots failing to pass the national inspection were frequently manufactured and in addition, the manufacturing technologies and quality control in those days did not reach satisfactory levels. The reason why the toxic material slipped through the national inspection remains unknown even now. It has been verified, however, that if random sampling had been performed properly, it is highly unlikely that toxic lots would have been overlooked.

The incident occurred in Shimane Prefecture soon after the occurrence in Kyoto Prefecture. In

製造したということから，薬事法違反で厚生省がトキソイドを製造した製薬会社を訴えました。結果として製薬会社の責任者は有罪となりましたが，大阪府から出向して，抜き取り検査を行った検査官は無罪となりました。また，当時の厚生省は被害者との裁判になれば敗訴になると判断して，補償金を早期に支払うことにより訴訟回避に動いたことが明らかになっています。戦後の日本でジフテリアが流行していたことがGHQの公衆衛生対策の直接のきっかけとされていますが，実際には，予防接種法が成立した1948年の時点でジフテリアの流行はほとんど終息に向かっていたのです。

ジフテリア予防接種禍事件に学ぶ

　この事件は戦後の占領下で発生したものです。当時の製造技術では安定した品質のトキソイド製造はできなかった状況でしたが，国家検定制度が形骸化していたことが直接の原因と考えられます。制度は容易に形骸化しうるものですが，品質チェックを最後の関門として全面的に依存するより，製造過程で品質を確保するということがまだ認識されない時代でした。京都府で被害が発生したのち，原因の究明を行わずに島根県で引き続き実施したため被害を拡大させてしまったことは，GHQの要請に従う形で拙速のまま予防接種を実施したことが背景として挙げられます。この事件では，国が被害者に見舞金を支払ったこともあって民事訴訟になりませんでしたが，国の医薬品行政，ことにワクチン行政が後年，国民の信頼を失う結果につながりました。

response to the Kyoto incident, the Ministry of Health and Welfare as well as the Shimane Prefectural Government at that time suspected that a particular lot was faulty, and judged that the other lots were safe, allowing the immunization be continued in Shimane Prefecture. In reality, however, the lots that were judged to be safe were defective since the national inspection was carelessly performed.

This incident caused a lawsuit, which was greatly different from court cases on sufferings induced by other drugs. The Ministry of Health and Welfare filed a criminal lawsuit against the manufacturer of the toxoid concerned on the grounds that the production company violated the Pharmaceutical Affairs Law; the trial resulted in verdicts of guilty for the responsible persons at the company and not guilty for the inspector performing sampling inspection who was temporarily assigned from the Osaka Prefectural Government. It was also revealed that the Ministry of Health and Welfare at that time paid financial compensation to the victims in early stages since they considered to lose a case filed by the victims and wanted to avoid lawsuits by paying compensation. The increasing number of cases of diphtheria in Japan in the post-war period was regarded as a direct cause for the GHQ to initiate the activities to control public health. In reality, however, at the time of the enactment of the Preventive Vaccination Law in 1948, the epidemic of diphtheria was coming to an end.

Lessons learned from the diphtheria immunization incident

This incident happened under the postwar occupation. Although the level of manufacturing technology at that time did not reach one of consistently producing toxoid of acceptable quality, the direct cause of this incident may be the fact that the national inspection system was turned into a mere formality. It is admitted, though, that any system can easily become a dead letter. In those days, a consensus was not yet established regarding the following point: product quality shall be secured not by totally relying on quality inspection as a final checkpoint but by performing stringent quality control checks throughout the manufacturing processes. The diphtheria immunization was continued in Shimane Prefecture even after the identification of victims in Kyoto Prefecture, without trying to determine the cause of the Kyoto incident, merely in accordance with the request by the GHQ, causing further expansion of the diphtheria tragedy. Although this incident led to no civil lawsuits partly because the national government paid financial compensation to the victims, it caused the general public to lose faith in drug administration, and the immunization program in particular, provided by the national government.

2 ペニシリンショック事件

事件の概要

　ペニシリンは細菌感染症に対する特効薬として米国で開発，実用化されました。日本においても，第二次世界大戦の末期には医薬品として実用化直前までの技術レベルに達していました。戦後は米国の指導や菌株の輸入などを通じて，ペニシリンが国産できるようになりました。その後，朝鮮戦争で増大した需要を賄うために生産量が増え，国民の手に届く医薬品となったのです。その効果は，1947年に肺炎で年間10万人が死亡しましたが，翌年にはその死亡者数が半減するほどでした。

　ペニシリンを製造するメーカーが多数(1955年当時，51社)になったことから販売競争も激化し，国民は容易にペニシリンを使えるようになりました。このため軽微な病気にもペニシリンが使われることとなり，ペニシリンに対する信頼も大きくなっていた時期にペニシリンショック事件が起きました。

　1956年，東京大学の教授が虫歯の治療のために化膿止めとしてペニシリンの注射を受け，5分もたたないうちにショック死しました。この事故は被害者が法曹界の重鎮であったことから，新聞に大きく報道されました。これをきっかけに，ペニシリンのショック死は，その年だけで40人以上の事故が明るみに出ました。その後，厚生省の調査により1953年から1957年の間に1,267人がショック症状を発現し，うち124人が死亡していることが明らかになっています。

　ペニシリンンに抗原性があることは，日本でショック死が社会問題化する前から米国ではすでに知られており，ペニシリンアレルギーについては，医師に対して警告と応急措置の用意が求められていました。日本では1951年ごろよりペニシリンアレルギーの研究が進み，1955年には厚生省はすでに40例あまりのペニシリンショック症例を収集していました。しかし，この情報は医療現場に活かされていませんでした。この事件をきっかけとして，ようやく問診や皮内反応テストの実施を添付文書に記載するようになりました。しかし，その後皮内テストではペニシリンアレルギーを十分予測できないことが明らかになり，アレルギーを含む既往歴の確認，救急処置の体制確保，投与開始から終了までの十分な観察をする方針に切り替わりました。今日，抗生物質によるショック死は激減しましたが，日本人にクスリ神話とクスリ恐怖神話の両方を残した事件でした。

2 Penicillin Shock Incident

Summary of the incident

Penicillin was developed and put into practical use as a specific medicine for bacterial infection in the US. Japan almost succeeded in commercialization of the drug as a pharmaceutical product soon before the end of World War II, after which Japan by itself became able to produce penicillin under directions given by the US and through import of the bacterial strains. Subsequently, the production quantity of the drug was increased to meet its increasing demand due to the Korean War, and the drug became available to the people. The effect was remarkable as indicated by reduction in deaths due to pneumonia to half in 1948 from 100,000 deaths in 1947.

Later, many manufacturers (51 as of 1955) produced penicillin, intensifying competition of sales of the drug and making the general public easier to use it. Under these circumstances, penicillin began to be used for even minor symptoms and the trust in the drug became greater. At that time, the penicillin shock incident occurred.

In 1956, a professor at The University of Tokyo received a penicillin injection during treatment of a decayed tooth for the purpose of preventing bacterial infection, and died in 5 minutes after the injection due to shock. Since the victim was a leading person in legal circles in Japan, this incident received prominent coverage in the newspapers. This news made known the fact that at least 40 persons had died due to penicillin shock only in that particular year. The subsequent survey by the Ministry of Health and Welfare revealed that during a period from 1953 to 1957, 1,267 persons experienced shock symptoms and 124 of them died.

In the US, it was already known that penicillin had antigenicity, and medical doctors were given warning against potential occurrence of penicillin allergy and requested to get emergency care prepared so that an adequate action was taken whenever necessary. These precautions were taken before the time at which the death due to penicillin shock became an issue of public concern in Japan. Research on penicillin allergy began to be active around in 1951 in Japan and the Ministry of Health and Welfare accumulated about 40 cases of penicillin shock in 1955. This information was not effectively utilized in actual clinical settings. The professor's death eventually made it mandatory to describe conduct of pre-treatment interview with patients and implementation of intradermal testing

ペニシリンショック事件に学ぶ

　ペニシリンは，戦後の日本の感染症治療を大きく変えた夢の薬剤でした。その治療効果にばかり目が奪われて，米国ではすでにとられていたペニシリンショックへの対応はとられていませんでした。事件を契機に厚生省は，アレルギーを含む既往歴の有無について問診を実施することとし，その結果，ペニシリンの副作用の可能性があるときは，他の治療法を選択するよう医療関係者に注意喚起を行いました。その後，薬剤の慎重な使用と救急措置体制の普及により，ペニシリンによる健康被害は激減しました。

in package inserts. However, the intradermal testing was later switched to the following policy since it became evident that with this testing, potential occurrence of penicillin allergy was not adequately foreseeable: confirmation of a history including allergy, establishment of a system for providing emergency care, and thorough observation from the start to the end of administration of penicillin. Since then, deaths due to shock caused by antibiotics declined sharply in Japan. The penicillin shock incident left both a myth about drugs and a myth about the fear of drugs in Japanese people.

Lessons learned from the penicillin shock incident

Penicillin was a dream medicine since it dramatically changed Japan's postwar treatment of infection. Its therapeutic effect was so impressive that it dazzled even the general population. No actions in response to penicillin shock were taken in Japan, although these actions had already been implemented in the US. This incident made the Ministry of Health and Welfare alert the healthcare professionals concerned to the following policy: to conduct pre-treatment interview with patients to confirm a history including allergy, and whenever the interview identifies a possibility of occurrence of a penicillin-related adverse reaction, to select another treatment. Subsequently, the careful use of drugs and the spread of systems for taking emergency care dramatically decreased health damage caused by penicillin.

3 サリドマイド事件

事件の概要

　サリドマイドによる胎児への健康被害は世界的な事件でした。日本においても，現在，309名の被害者がいます（2013年時点で）。日本におけるサリドマイド事件の最大の特徴は，被害拡大を防ぐ機会を適切にとらえて対応していれば，被害者数をもっと抑えられたであろうということです。

　サリドマイド製剤は，わが国でも海外と同様に安全な睡眠薬として，1958年に発売されました。さらに1960年には胃腸薬にも配合され，多くの薬品として市販されました。日本では1959年から被害者が誕生し始めました。サリドマイドの開発会社であるグリュネンタール社は，日本の製薬企業にレンツ警告を1961年に届けました。翌1962年，日本の製薬企業は社員を西ドイツに派遣しましたが，正確な情報は日本にもたらされませんでした。さらにグリュネンタール社は，その後2回にわたって日本の製薬企業に販売中止の警告を届けていました。しかし，日本の行政当局と製薬企業の反応ははかばかしいものではありませんでした。

　製薬企業のみならず一部の学者も，日本には胎芽病というものはないと主張していました。サリドマイドによる障害は胎児の器官形成期，すなわち各器官が"芽"の時期に傷害を及ぼすため，"胎芽病"といわれています。しかし小児科学会で胎芽病発生の発表が新聞報道されると，1962年9月，製薬企業は因果関係を否定しながらもサリドマイド製剤の市場からの回収に踏み切りました。西ドイツの決定から10か月後の対応となりました。しかもその回収は不徹底なものでした。このため1963年，1964年，1969年と被害者の誕生が続きました。西ドイツの決定から遅れることなく，また徹底した回収が行われていれば，多くの子供たちが被害を受けずにすんだともいわれています。

　日本での被害が一層悲惨なものとなったのは，社会の偏見と差別でした。サリドマイド被害児の生存率は欧米で60～80％とされているのに対し，日本ではわずかに20～25％です。しかも日本の被害児より，欧米での被害児の症状が重いのです。この数字は，日本では被害児の多くが出生しなかったか，死産として扱われた可能性が高いことを示唆しています。

3 Thalidomide Incident

Summary of the incident

The thalidomide-caused damage to fetuses was a worldwide tragedy. In Japan, 309 victims survive as of 2013. The greatest feature of the thalidomide-induced suffering in Japan was that if an opportunity to prevent expansion of the damage had been identified properly so as to take adequate actions to prevent further expansion, the number of victims would have been significantly reduced.

In 1958, a thalidomide pharmaceutical was launched as a safe sleeping pill, as in foreign countries, onto the Japanese market. In 1960, thalidomide was combined with other ingredients in many medications for the digestive organs and thus was further available commercially. Starting in 1959, thalidomide victims were born in Japan. In 1961, Grünenthal, the company that developed thalidomide, provided a warning by Prof. W. Lenz to the marketing company of the drug in Japan, and in 1962, the Japanese marketing company dispatched its staff to West Germany, although no accurate information was delivered to Japan. Following this, Grünenthal delivered twice the warning to discontinue marketing of the drug to the Japanese marketer. However, the regulatory authorities in Japan and the Japanese marketer did not make a prompt response to these warnings.

Not only the pharmaceutical companies but also some experts claimed that a disease called embryopathy did not exist in Japan. Deformities caused by thalidomide developed in the embryonic period, during which organogenesis occurs, and had impact on the embryo; these congenital anomalies are called "embryopathies". Press reporting that the embryopathy was presented at a Japanese scientific meeting forced the Japanese marketing company to decide to initiate recall of the thalidomide preparation from the market in September 1962, although they denied a causal relationship between the disease and the drug. The recall in Japan happened 10 months after the recall of the drug in West Germany, and was not adequately conducted, resulting in continuous births of thalidomide victims in 1963, 1964, and 1969. For this reason it is estimated that if the drug had been withdrawn adequately and thoroughly from the Japanese market immediately after the decision was made in West Germany, many of the thalidomide cases would have been prevented.

Prejudice and discrimination in society against thalidomide-related birth deformities further increased the severity of thalidomide tragedy in Japan. The survival rate of thalidomide victims is

この事件について，被害者は当初法務局への人権侵害の申し立てを行い，製薬企業に補償を求めましたがいずれも受け入れられず，1963年に訴訟となりました。薬害に関して日本初の民事訴訟でした。この訴訟では一部の著名な学者や専門家が，サリドマイド原因説を否定したり，サリドマイドは一要因にすぎないと主張したり，さらにはレンツの調査に誤りがあると意図的に歪曲した解説を述べる等，製薬企業を擁護した主張をしました。

　裁判は，グリュネンタール社が西ドイツで被害補償を提示したことから，厚生省と製薬企業は安全性の確認とレンツ警告への対応に落ち度があったことを認め，1972年に和解が成立しました。提訴してから10年後のことでした。

サリドマイド事件に学ぶ

　サリドマイド事件当時の日本の薬事法は，戦後の混乱期を乗り切るために1948年に制定された旧薬事法を基に，1960年に制定された薬事法でした。その立法趣旨は，医薬品の製造・輸入販売行為を規制することに重点が置かれていました。これは当時の世界の趨勢で，現在のように医薬品の有効性と安全性をデータに基づいて適切に評価することはなく，海外情報を系統的に収集・評価して承認審査や市販後の安全対策に活かすということも行われていませんでした。なによりも，薬の安全性について関係者や一般国民の関心は高くなかったのです。

　この事件の教訓として，次のような対策が取られました。

1. 新薬の申請要件の見直し

　1) 胎児に対する影響に関する動物試験法を定め，従来の基礎的試験資料に加えて申請書の添付資料とすることになりました。

　2) 臨床試験については，二重盲検法等による客観性の高い資料及び従来の臨床施設2か

estimated to be 60% to 80% in European and North American countries, whereas it is as low as 20% to 25% in Japan. In addition, the extent of deformities of victims are more severe in European and North American countries than in Japan. These figures suggest that many of the victims in Japan were not born or handled as stillbirths.

The thalidomide victims first brought accusations of human rights violations at the Regional Legal Affairs Bureau and claimed compensatory damages from the pharmaceutical company concerned. Neither of them was accepted, and the victims and their families filed a civil lawsuit in 1963. This was the first lawsuit involving drug-induced suffering in Japan. In this litigation, some influential researchers and experts ruled out the belief that thalidomide caused the birth deformities concerned or claimed that thalidomide was merely a single factor in the occurrence of these adverse health effects. Some even gave an intentionally distorted explanation by saying that there were mistakes in the study by Prof. W. Lenz. These allegations were in favor of the Japanese marketing company.

The tide of the litigation was changed by the fact that Grünenthal in West Germany agreed to pay financial compensation to the children with malformations attributable to thalidomide. The Japanese Ministry of Health and Welfare and the marketing company admitted that they had not adequately confirmed safety and properly responded to Lenz's warning. A formal settlement was made in 1972, almost 10 years after the lawsuit was first filed.

Lessons learned from the thalidomide incident

The Pharmaceutical Affairs Law (PAL) in Japan that was effective at the time of the thalidomide incident was established in 1960, but it was based on the Old PAL enacted in 1948 with the intention of getting through the postwar turmoil. The then PAL placed importance on regulatory control of manufacture, import, and marketing of drugs, which was consistent with the world trend at that time. Neither proper review of drugs based on data regarding safety and efficacy nor systemic collection and evaluation of overseas information so as to make the best use of such information on approval reviews and post-marketing safety management were performed then. There was also a low level of interest in drug safety among the people concerned and the general public.

The thalidomide tragedy facilitated reshaping of drug administration in Japan as described below.

1. Review of requirements for approval review for new drugs

1) The methods for conducting animal studies to evaluate effects on fetuses were defined, and it was required to include data from studies conducted in accordance with these methods, in

所，60例以上という基準をはるかに上回る症例数を要求することになりました。
3) 新薬の前臨床試験における吸収・分布・代謝・排泄に関する資料の重要性が認識されて，その資料の添付を要求することになりました。

2. 医薬品の製造承認等に関する基本方針

従来慣行的に行われてきた方針を集大成し，体系的に明確にするとともに新しい方針を加えて「医薬品の製造承認等に関する基本方針」を定めて，薬務局長通知で関係方面に通知しました。この方針は1999年に大幅に改定されるまで，30年余りにわたって新薬承認審査の基本として運用されてきました。

医薬品の製造承認等に関する基本方針（1967年）

・申請資料の明確化
　—医薬品の製造承認申請等に添付する資料の範囲を医薬品の区分に応じて明確化
・医療用医薬品と一般用医薬品の区分の導入
　—医薬品を医療用医薬品と一般用医薬品に区分し，それぞれの特性を考慮した承認審査を行うこととした
・医療用配合剤の明確化
　—原則として，配合理由がすでに学問的に確立しているものであって，用時調整が困難なもの，又は配合理由として副作用の軽減又は相乗効果があることが立証されているもの（1999年，2005年に配合剤の範囲は拡大された）に限ったこと
・新開発医薬品の副作用報告
　—新開発医薬品の製造承認を受けた企業は，承認を受けた日から少なくとも2年間，副作用に関する情報を報告すること

addition to data of basic studies which was already a requirement, in approval applications.

2) For clinical trials, data of greater objectivity obtained by double-blind methodology or any other relevant methods was required. In addition, the required number of patients in a clinical trial was made much higher than the previous standard, i.e. at least 60 patients in at least 2 medical institutions.

3) The importance of data regarding absorption, distribution, metabolism, and excretion of a new drug in pre-clinical studies was recognized, and it was required to submit such data with approval applications.

2. Basic Policy on Approval for Manufacture, etc. of Drugs

The Notification entitled "Basic Policy on Approval for Manufacture, etc. of Drugs", which compiled the policies that had so far been the customary practices, organized them in a systemic and definite manner, and which included new policies, was issued by the Director-General of Pharmaceutical Affairs Bureau, Ministry of Health and Welfare in 1967. This Basic Policy was applied to approval review for new drugs for more than 30 years until a substantial amendment was made to the Policy in 1999.

Basic Policy on Approval for Manufacture, etc. of Drugs (1967)

- **Clarification of data to be submitted with approval applications**
  —The scope of data to be submitted with approval applications, etc. for manufacture of drugs was defined according to drug classifications.
- **Introduction of categories of prescription and non-prescription drugs**
  —The drugs were divided into two categories, i.e. prescription drugs and non-prescription drugs. It was required to take the individual features when conducting approval review.
- **Clarification of combination prescription drugs**
  —The combination prescription drug was defined as those for which as a rule the rationale for combination had already been established on the basis of scientific studies and in addition, preparation of the drug by combining relevant ingredients before every use was difficult, or for which it had been proved that the combination of ingredients concerned relieved adverse drug reactions or produced synergic effects. (Note that the scope of definition of combination drugs was enlarged in 1999 and 2005.)
- **Adverse drug reaction reporting for newly developed drugs**
  —A company who obtained an approval for manufacture of a newly developed drug was required to report information regarding adverse reactions of the drug for at least 2 years since the day on which the approval was granted to the company.

4 アンプル入り風邪薬事件

事件の概要

　アンプル入り風邪薬とは，風邪薬を液剤としてアンプルに封入したもので，薬局で買える一般用医薬品として発売されました。成分は解熱鎮痛成分であるアミノピリン，スルピリンを主体として，ビタミンなどを加えたものでした。この事件が社会問題化する以前から，1回の常用量を超える成分を含有するアンプル製剤が販売されていたため，厚生省は1964年，アンプル入り内服液の用法を1回1容器として服用できる範囲に制限していました。アンプル入り風邪薬の成分は従来の風邪薬と違ったところはありませんでしたが，注射薬の即効性をイメージした商品でした。

　この事件は，高度成長時代を背景とした1965年のA型インフルエンザ流行のさなかに発生しました。当時，インフルエンザによる患者数は2万6,000人，学級閉鎖は2,400校に上りました。薬局の店頭で，効き目がすぐ出ると宣伝されたアンプル入り風邪薬を一気に飲んで，仕事に向かうというのがそのころの風潮でした。1965年2月に発生した死亡事故は，解熱剤として処方されていたピリン系薬物（アミノピリンやスルピリンなど）によるアレルギー性のショックでした。このアレルギーで死亡する消費者が続出したことをきっかけに，各地でアンプル入り風邪薬の死亡事故が相次いで報道されました。この健康被害は当初，患者の特異体質が原因であるとされていましたが，社会問題化したために1962年，厚生省はアンプル入り風邪薬の広告・販売の中止を業界に申し入れをしました。

　一部の製薬企業は長年の実績を持っていたことから，死亡事故は偶然が重なったためであり，また厚生省の基準に従って製造したのであるから，と難色を示しましたが，最終的には各社が販売停止に応じました。しかし販売停止にはなったものの市場からの回収は行わなかったために，ショック死はその後も続発しました。そのため厚生省は，1965年3月に市場からの回収を要請し，各社は「回収及び返品に伴う損失を補填する優遇措置」を条件にこれを受け入れました。つまり税制，金融上の優遇，剤形変更に伴う承認許可の優遇でした。これにより市場から3,000万本のアンプル入り風邪薬が回収されました。

　厚生省の対応は英断と評価されましたが，回収が終わった時点で製薬会社を集め，製薬業界に損害を与えたことを陳謝しました。製薬企業に対するこの配慮が，後のクロロキンによる網膜症被害への対応の遅れにつながったとされます。この事件を契機に，日本製薬

4 Cold-Medicines-in-Ampoules Incident

Summary of the incident

Cold-medicines-in-ampoules were manufactured by sealing cold medicines in liquid form into ampoules, and were marketed as over-the-counter drugs at pharmacies. The ampoule contained an antipyretic and analgesic drug such as aminopyrine or sulpyrine as a main active ingredient and also vitamins. Before the deaths from shock caused by cold medicines in ampoules became an issue of public concern in 1965, ampoules containing the active ingredient at a dose higher than its usual dose per administration had been marketed. In 1964, the Ministry of Health and Welfare (MHW) imposed limitations on the administration of oral liquid medicines in ampoules; only one ampoule containing the usual dose of the drug was allowed per dosing. The active ingredients contained in these ampoules were the same as those already used in existing cold remedies. This product delivered an image of rapid effectiveness, just like injections.

When this drug-induced suffering became the focus of public concern in 1965, there had been an epidemic of influenza type A affecting 26,000 people. Because of the epidemic, 2,400 schools throughout Japan temporarily suspended classes. At that time, Japan was in the middle of nearly two decades of rapid economic growth sustained by the efforts of hard working people. Even though they had a touch of slight cold, workers would not take time off. Instead they would buy cold-medicines-in-ampoules, which were advertised to be rapidly effective, quickly consumed them on the spot at the pharmacy, and then went off to work. This was the trend at that time. In February 1965, some individuals who consumed cold-medicines-in-ampoules died, and the deaths were caused by allergic shock due to pyrine preparations (such as aminopyrine and sulpyrine) prescribed as antipyretics. The deaths in succession due to the allergy triggered reporting through the mass media of deaths caused by cold-medicines-in-ampoules across Japan. It was initially suspected that this health damage might have been related to idiosyncrasy. However, since this became a social issue, the MHW requested the industry to discontinue the advertisement and marketing of such cold-medicines-in-ampoules in 1962.

Some of the pharmaceutical companies expressed reluctance to accept the request, claiming that considering their long-term business performance, these deaths resulted from a combination of coincidences, and that they manufactured the ampoules in accordance with the standards

団体連合会は医薬品広告に関する自主規制を行い，医薬品の宣伝量が急速に減少しました。

アンプル入り風邪薬事件に学ぶ

　アンプル入り風邪薬は液剤であったために吸収が速く，毒性も著しく強く発現するという薬理学的には当然予想される製剤設計上の問題を含んでいました。それに加えて，薬理作用の強い成分や一回用量以上に成分が配合された製品もありました。このため，配合剤に対する安全性を十分に検討した承認審査の必要性が認識され，中央薬事審議会に配合剤調査会が新設されました。

　販売においては，高度経済成長期に人々は長時間にわたり仕事をして，少しの不調は薬で手軽に治すという風潮を背景に，乱用を助長する製薬企業の宣伝広告も行われていました。本書では取り上げていませんが，1980年代に麻薬成分を含有する鎮咳去痰剤の若者への販売が社会問題化したことがあります。薬は乱用されることがあり，医薬品の宣伝広告は適正使用を促す，抑制のきいたものでなければなりません。

prescribed by the MHW. Eventually, the companies all accepted the request of discontinuation of marketing. They stopped marketing the ampoules but unfortunately did not retrieve the products from the market, and deaths due to shock continued to occur. In March 1965, the MHW requested the pharmaceutical companies concerned to retrieve the products from the market, and the companies accepted this request on the condition that they received "preferential treatment to compensate for losses caused by the recalls and returned products". This meant tax incentives, financial relief, and preferential treatment to obtain official approvals for change in dosage forms. As a result of this, thirty million ampoules containing cold medicines were retrieved from the market.

The decision made by the MHW was widely considered to be wise and appropriate. However, after completion of the recalls, the MHW gathered the pharmaceutical companies together, and extended them a profound apology for damages caused due to the withdrawal. It is possible that this withdrawal and the repercussions within the industry would later lead to hesitation and weakness on the part of the MHW in taking future action against pharmaceutical companies. For example, it appears that the regulatory authority delayed in taking responsive actions to retinopathy caused by chloroquine, another drug-induced suffering that occurred in later years. The cold-medicines-in-ampoules incident encouraged the Federation of Pharmaceutical Manufacturers' Associations of Japan to put voluntary restraints on advertisements of drugs, and as a result, drug advertising declined sharply.

Lessons learned from the cold-medicines-in-ampoules incident

The cold-medicines-in-ampoules had some problems relating to its formulation that were reasonably foreseeable from the viewpoint of pharmacology: they were in liquid dosage form and thus, rapidly absorbed, causing remarkably strong toxicity. In addition, some of the ampoule products contained combinations of drugs having strong pharmacological effects and others contained an active ingredient at a dose greater than its defined dose per administration. This incident contributed to raising people's awareness over the safety of combination drugs, and the need for thorough evaluation through approval reviews. As a result, the Subcommittee of Combination Drugs was newly established in the Central Pharmaceutical Affairs Council.

During the period of Japan's rapid economic growth, there was a trend across the nation where people dedicated themselves to jobs and denied their own health. Workers would treat minor illness by taking convenient, over-the-counter remedies, under which some advertisements by pharmaceutical companies may have prompted overuse and even abuse of drugs. Although not described in this book, in the 1980s, the sale of cough medicines containing narcotics to young people became an issue of public concern. Since drugs may be abused, advertisements on drugs

must promote their proper use and be reasonably regulated.

5 スモン事件

事件の概要

　SMONとはSubacute Myelo-Optico-Neuropathy（亜急性脊髄視神経症）の略称です。この症状は下痢や腹痛などの消化器症状に引き続いて，足裏の激しいしびれ，激痛，運動麻痺などが上肢へと上がってきます。時に失明，排尿障害，発汗障害，性機能障害などを伴う全身に及ぶ難治性疾患です。現在でも根治療法はないとされます。

　スモン事件は，日本でも戦前から使われていたキノホルムという薬が原因です。最初の症例は1958年に学会報告されました。このときは多発性神経炎様症状として報告されましたが，後にSMONと命名されました。以後，この健康被害は1967年から1968年にかけて全国で多発し，最終的には約15年の長きに亘って被害者が発生しました。厚生省が認定した被害者は10,007名，推定では12,000名から16,000名に上るとされています。しかし，実態はこの3倍以上だとする研究者もいます。

　日本では，キノホルムは1936年にアメーバ赤痢の治療薬として劇薬に指定され，投与の上限量や投与期間について厳しい制限の下で使用されていました。その後，1939年の戦時薬局方において，アメーバ赤痢のほか各種の細菌性及び寄生虫性腸疾患，異常発酵，腸チフスあるいは熱帯地方腸障害などへの適応が拡大され，用法用量も大幅に緩和された上，劇薬指定が解除されました。戦後，キノホルムは180種もの一般用胃腸薬に配合され，販売されました。製薬企業は一般の下痢，腸疾患の薬，整腸保健薬として大々的にプロモーションを行いました。

　この健康被害の原因について行政も研究班を組織して対応しましたが，容易に原因はわかりませんでした。この間，巷では奇病，伝染病との評判が立ち，また一部の研究者もウイルス説を主張しました。このため，治療法のない伝染病に罹患したとされる被害者やその家族が過酷な差別や偏見によって，自殺や安楽死に追い込まれたという悲劇が少なからず起きたのです。これは薬害の二次被害というべきものでした。

　この事件は，キノホルムが鉄とのキレートを作ってスモン患者の尿に緑色の結晶を析出することが偶然に発見され，それをきっかけとした疫学的調査により，原因がキノホルムであるとする手がかりが得られました。行政はこの手がかりを得た2か月後の1970年9月

5 | SMON Incident

Summary of the incident

SMON is an abbreviation for subacute myelo-optico-neuropathy. It is a refractory disease with systemic effects; gastrointestinal symptoms such as diarrhea and abdominal pain, followed by severe numbness and tingling in the soles of feet that eventually turns into total loss of sensation and then paralysis of the feet and legs. Sometimes, blindness, micturition disturbance, perspiration disorders, and sexual dysfunction occur. Even as of today, there is no radical treatment for the disease.

SMON was caused by clioquinol, a drug which had been used long from before World War II in Japan. The first patient was reported as a case of multiple neuritis-like symptoms at a general scientific meeting of a Japanese society in 1958. This disease was later named SMON. In 1967 to 1968, a large number of Japanese citizens were afflicted with this disease and eventually, SMON victims were identified over a period of as long as about 15 years. The Ministry of Health and Welfare certified 10,007 patients as SMON victims, although the generally estimated number totals between 12,000 and 16,000. Some researchers believe that the real number of victims is more than 3 times greater than the above-stated figures.

In 1936 in Japan, clioquinol was designated by the Minister of Health and Welfare as a powerful drug indicated for the treatment of amoebic dysentery. The drug was therefore used with severe limitations posed on the highest dose and length of treatment. In 1939, the wartime Japanese Pharmacopoeia expanded its indications to the treatment of, among others, various types of bacterial and parasitic bowel diseases, abnormal fermentation of intestinal contents, typhoid, and bowel disorders of tropical countries; furthermore it substantially relieved the limitations on dosage and administration, and withdrew the designation of powerful drug. After the end of World War II, clioquinol was combined with other ingredients in as many as 180 over-the-counter (OTC) combination drugs for the digestive organs which were marketed in Japan. The responsible pharmaceutical companies extensively conducted promotional activities of clioquinol for common diarrhea, bowel diseases, and all types of abdominal disturbances.

In time the Japanese government organized a study group to try to identify possible causes of the

に販売及び使用の中止を決定しました。キノホルムの販売中止によって，スモン発症者は1971年に36名，1972年2名，1973年1名，以後発症者はゼロとなりました。

　スモン事件は1971年の損害賠償請求訴訟を皮切りに，全国で33の地方裁判所と8つの高等裁判所で争われ，原告は7,561人に膨れ上がりました。裁判では最後までウイルス説に固執した製薬企業があり，裁判は長期化しました。原告が各地の地裁で勝訴を積み重ねる中で，1979年9月に国と主要な被告企業3社が責任を認めて和解に至りました。最初の症例が報告されてから21年後のことでした。地裁での勝訴判決趣旨はそれぞれ異なりますが，1979年8月の前橋判決では「医薬品は不可欠な財であるが一般の患者はその安全性を確認する手段を持たない上に，医薬品製造業者が利益追求のあまり安全性確保の履行をなおざりにする可能性がある。公正な立場と高度の技術と組織を有しうる国が医薬品の安全性確保に関与することは国民にとって極めて必要性が高い」と，国の責任を認めました。

　この薬害事件をきっかけに，訴訟とは別に患者救済を目的として医薬品副作用被害救済基金法が成立しました。この法律に基づき1980年の5月から救済制度が施行されました。今日，裁判で和解したスモン被害者に対しては，医薬品医療機器総合機構が原因企業の委託を受けて，健康管理手当および介護費用の支払い業務を代行しています。

adverse health effects of clioquinol, but these were not immediately identified. In the meantime, the spreading rumor was that SMON was a bizarre or communicable disease. Some researchers proposed that the disease was caused by a virus. Under these circumstances, there was an accumulation of unreasonably wrong perceptions that victims had an untreatable disease which might be communicable to others, leading to tragic events in no small numbers: both victims and their family members suffered under harsh discrimination and prejudice, resulting in case of suicide and euthanasia. These should be regarded as secondary tragedies to drug-induced sufferings.

Nurses coincidentally discovered that the urine of SMON patients was green. Subsequent epidemiological surveys found that clioquinol chelated with ferric iron and the iron chelate was identified as the green substance in the urine of SMON patients. These survey results attributed SMON to clioquinol. In September 1970, two months after the attribution, the Japanese government decided to ban marketing and use of the drug in Japan. Because of this decision, the number of patients who newly suffered from SMON was reduced to 36 in 1971, 2 in 1972, one in 1973, and no more thereafter.

The first lawsuit for claiming compensatory damages due to SMON was filed in 1971, followed by additional ones brought in 33 district courts and 8 high courts throughout Japan. Eventually, the plaintiffs totaled 7,561. Since one of the defendant companies refused to give up the allegedly proposed virus-causing belief in the trials, the trials continued for a long time. As the plaintiffs won the lawsuits one after another at the level of the district courts, the national government and the major 3 defendant companies admitted their liabilities and reached settlements in court, which was 21 years after reporting of the first patient. The point of the adjudication in favor of the plaintiff at the district courts varied depending on the judges. The Maebashi District Court recognized the liability of the Japanese government by making the following judgment in August 1979: "Although drugs are essential assets, ordinary patients usually do not have measures to confirm the safety of drugs and in addition, drug manufacturers may be highly likely to neglect implementation of activities to secure the drug safety since they put too much importance on seeking profits. The national government shall deal with such situations from a fair standpoint and can possess advanced technologies and organizations, and thus, the national government's involvement in securing drug safety is an extremely great need for the people".

The SMON incident not only resulted in the lawsuits but also prompted the establishment of the "Act on Adverse Drug Reaction Relief Services Fund" for the purpose of providing relief for sufferers from drug adverse reactions, under which the Relief System for Adverse Drug Reactions was started in May 1980. At present, the Pharmaceuticals and Medical Devices Agency provides healthcare allowances and nursing care expenses to the SMON victims who agreed upon

スモン事件に学ぶ

　キノホルム製剤は昔から使われていましたが，使い方や用法用量，適応症が変わることにより新たなリスクが生じました。最初は外用剤であったものが内服薬となり，適応症が拡がり，用法用量も拡大し，大量，長期連用とリスク要因を重ねてしまった結果がスモン事件を生み出しました。医薬品の適応症が拡がることは有用性も拡大することですが，リスクも同時に拡大する可能性もあると言えます。この点において，審査及び安全対策の在り方は極めて重要です。

　スモン事件のもう一つの問題提起は，薬害における被害者救済でした。薬害は短期間に多数の被害者を発生させうること，裁判で争うには知識，専門性，費用，投薬証明などあらゆる面において被害者(原告)は不利な立場にあること，また損害賠償訴訟においては被告(国，企業，医師など)の過失を証明する必要があるなど負担の多いものでした。その結果，裁判での決着は長期間にわたり，被害者の負担はますます過大なものとなります。これらのことから，訴訟を起こす権利とは別に1979年に「医薬品副作用被害救済基金」が設立され，1980年から救済業務が開始されました。

　この「医薬品副作用被害救済制度」の導入と並んで，1979年に薬事法が大幅かつ全面的に改正されました。以下に示した改正は，現在の薬事制度の枠組みとして生きています。

・従来は行政指導であった承認基準と承認に必要な資料が明確化されました
・日本薬局方収載医薬品についても原則として承認を要することとなりました。
・承認6年後に再審査を行う再審査制度が導入されました。
・従来は行政指導であった再評価制度が法制化されました。
・従来は行政指導であった医薬品の副作用情報の収集，提供，報告に関する規定が法制化されました。
・従来は行政指導であったGMPが法制化されました。
・医薬品による健康被害拡大のおそれのある時に，販売の一時停止や回収等緊急措置命令の権限が明確化されました。
・添付文書に禁忌，副作用等の記載が義務化されました。
・医薬品の安全性について虚偽または誇大な広告が禁止されました。

settlements in the trial, under commission from the drug manufacturers liable for causing SMON in such patients.

Lessons learned from the SMON incident

Even though clioquinol products had been long used, changes in the method of use, dosage and administration, or indications resulted in new risks. The drug was originally developed as topical preparations, but then started to be taken orally and the indications gradually extended. Dosage and administration were expanded, resulting in their use at larger doses for longer periods of time. The accumulation of these risks led to the SMON incident. Extension of indications of a drug typically means enlargement of the area of its usefulness, although such extension is simultaneously associated with potentially expanding risks. It is therefore critical for the regulatory authorities to carefully review drugs with such potential taken into account prior to granting approval for marketing and also to closely watch its use in postmarketing phase with special regard to risk minimization.

Another byproduct of the SMON incident was the establishment of the relief system for victims of drug-induced sufferings. Once a drug-induced suffering occurs, not a small number of victims can be identified in a short period of time. If victims, who are usually non-professionals, are going to file a lawsuit in a court of law, they (the plaintiff) have to bear great burdens: they are handicapped in all aspects relating to the disputed issue(s), including, among others, knowledge, specialty, required costs, and demonstrating that treatment with the drug concerned was actually administered, and in lawsuits for claiming damage compensation, they must prove the negligence of the defendant (e.g. the national government, companies, and/or medical doctors). Consequently, trials continue for a prolonged time of period, which causes victims to bear further greater burdens. In addition to the right to file lawsuits that victims have, the "Fund for Relief Services for Adverse Drug Reactions" was established in 1979 and the relief services for sufferers from drug adverse reactions were started in 1980.

Along with the introduction of the "Relief System for Adverse Drug Reactions", the Pharmaceutical Affairs Law underwent a major amendment in 1979 as indicated below. This amendment forms an essential framework of the currently valid drug administration in Japan.
- Clarification of both approval criteria and data required for approval (Both of them had formerly been subject to administrative guidance, which has no legal binding force.)
- Approval required, in principle, for articles included in the Japanese Pharmacopoeia
- Introduction of the reexamination system for reexamination at 6 years after approval of a new drug

- Legalization of the reevaluation system for drugs (formerly administrative guidance)
- Legalization of specifications for collection, provision, and reporting of information on adverse drug reactions (formerly administrative guidance)
- Legalization of GMP (formerly administrative guidance)
- Clarification of the authority to place orders for emergency measures such as temporary discontinuation of marketing or recalls when health damage due to a drug may expand
- Obligation to enter contraindications, adverse drug reactions, etc. in package inserts of drugs
- Prohibition of false or misleading advertising of the safety of drugs

6 筋短縮症事件

事件の概要

　この事件の健康被害は，筋肉注射のために筋肉が永続的な萎縮を生じるものです。この萎縮の症状は，最初に山梨県という日本の中央部に位置する一地区で発見されました。1973年にこの地区で行われた3歳児検診で，歩き方の不自然な子供が多数発見されたことがきっかけとなって，事件として表面化しました。この集団発生については，東京大学の若手の有志の医師が中心となった自主検診団が調査に当たりました。その結果，171名の小児のうち130名に異常が見られました。そしてこの健康被害は頻回の筋肉注射が原因で，しかも地区の特定の医院での注射が原因であることが強く疑われました。

　この調査報告は新聞などのメディアで全国に報じられました。すると，1963年には静岡県で，1969年には福井県で，また1970年には愛知県でも集団発生していることが明らかになりました。これらの健康被害は，それまで偶発的な医療ミスとして扱われており，薬害として認識されていませんでした。その後，自主検診団の調査と厚生省の調査を合わせて，患者数は約2万人となりました。しかし集団検診を実施すれば必ずこのような筋肉の萎縮症状が発見されたことから，全国で10万人規模の被害であろうと推定されました。

　健康被害は注射の部位によって，大腿四頭筋短縮症，臀筋短縮症，三角筋短縮症及び腕三頭筋短縮症と呼ばれていましたが，現在では筋短縮症として統一されています。筋肉注射により筋肉が繊維状に変化し，弾力を失った結果，子供の成長によって伸びる骨格にそって筋肉が伸びることができないため，関節が曲がりにくくなります。そのため，動作が制限されて，動きが不自然になってしまうのです。

　筋肉注射の回数と萎縮症状の程度はおおむね比例しており，数十回から100回以上の注射をされた被害者も多くいました。しかし，神経に近いところへ注射された場合には，数回の注射で短縮症になったケースも発見されています。注射の適用となったもともとの症状は，風邪や下痢などの比較的軽度のものでした。注射された薬剤は抗生物質や解熱剤，ビタミン剤などでした。当時は点滴などの注射技術がなく，また患者の両親も注射をありがたがる風潮がありました。

　日本では1946年，筋短縮症が日本整形外科学会で報告されましたが，その後も症例報

6 Muscle Contracture Incident

Summary of the incident

The damage to health in this incident was permanent muscle contracture caused by intramuscular injection. The contracture related symptoms were first discovered in a district in Yamanashi Prefecture, a less industrialized province notable for its mountains, lakes and valleys. In 1973, the free health checkups for 3-year-old infants that were provided by the municipality of this district revealed abnormal walking patterns in many children, which first brought this outbreak to public attention. A voluntary medical checkup group consisting mainly of young medical doctors at The University of Tokyo investigated children in this district and found abnormalities in 130 of 171 children they examined. It was strongly suspected that this suffering might have been caused by frequent intramuscular injections at a particular clinic in this district.

The investigation results were reported throughout Japan by the mass media such as newspapers, which further discovered epidemics of the same suffering in Shizuoka Prefecture in 1963, in Fukui Prefecture in 1969, and in Aichi Prefecture in 1970. These cases were handled as incidental medical malpractices and were not recognized as the drug-induced suffering. Subsequent surveys by both the voluntary medical checkup group and the Ministry of Health and Welfare discovered a total of about 20,000 patients. The total number of victims throughout Japan was estimated to be closer to 100,000 since each implementation of health checkup discovered without fail the symptoms due to muscle contracture.

The suffering was named differently depending on injection sites as follows: quadriceps contracture (injection in the thigh), gluteus contracture (in the buttock), deltoid contracture (in the shoulder), and triceps contracture (in the arm). They are currently unified to a single name of muscle contracture. Intramuscular injection causes fibrous change in muscles, resulting in loss of elasticity of the affected muscles. As children grow up, their bones elongate but their affected muscles cannot stretch completely, causing joints to get hard to bend; the movement is restricted and becomes abnormal.

The number of intramuscular injections was almost proportional to the severity of symptoms. In many of the victims, the number of injections per patient ranged from several tens to 100's or more.

告が続きました。1973年に山梨県での集団発生が発見されたときにはすでに，540例の学会報告が積みあがっていました。しかしこの情報は，小児科関連の学会や一般臨床医家には共有されていませんでした。このため健康被害が社会問題化したあと，日本整形外科学会と日本小児科学会はこの健康被害を防止できなかったことについて反省の声明文を出すことになりました。

　この事件は全国で訴訟となりました。被告は国，製薬会社，医師・病院と，日本医師会でした。裁判は18年の長期に亘った末，各地で和解決着しました。請求額に比べてほど遠い金額で和解せざるを得ませんでした。

筋短縮症事件に学ぶ

　筋肉注射の危険性は，海外では既に知られており，また国内でも一部の研究者には知られていました。しかし，一般臨床医家の間には浸透していませんでした。筋短縮症を生んだ筋肉注射は小児科，産科，内科などの医師が行い，筋短縮症の治療は整形外科医が担当しましたが，その両者での連携や情報交換が十分でなかったことが挙げられます。したがって，学会や日本医師会などの職能団体の果たす役割も十分ではありませんでした。この点を踏まえて日本小児科学会が1976年に以下の提言を発表し，関係学会にも周知しました。

・注射は親の要求ではなく，医師の医学的判断により行う
・風邪(症候群)には注射を極力避ける
・経口投与が可能であれば注射を避ける
・抗生物質と他剤との混注を避ける
・皮下への大量注射は行わない

　この提言により，今日では注射はできるだけ控えるようになりました。

In some patients whose injection sites were closer to nerves, muscle contracture developed only after several administrations. These intramuscular injections were used to deliver antibiotics, antipyretics, and vitamins for the purpose of treating relatively mild symptoms such as common cold and diarrhea. In those days, no other injecting technology, e.g. drip infusion, was available and patients' parents tended to value injections very much.

In Japan, muscle contracture was reported at a scientific meeting of the Japanese Orthopedic Association in 1946 and following this, additional case reports continued to be presented. When the epidemic in Yamanashi Prefecture was discovered in 1973, 540 patients had already been reported at scientific conferences relating to orthopedics. This information was not shared with scientific associations relating to pediatrics or general clinicians. After this health damage attracted public attention and became a social issue, the Japanese Orthopedic Association and the Japan Pediatric Society issued their statements indicating that they felt sorry about their failure to prevent the health damage.

This incident brought about lawsuits across Japan and the defendants included the national government, pharmaceutical companies, medical doctors, hospitals, and the Japan Medical Association. The trials lasted for as long as 18 years and eventually, the plaintiffs had to admit settlement at much smaller amounts of money than what they claimed for in compensatory damages.

Lessons learned from the muscle contracture incident

The risks associated with intramuscular injection had been known outside Japan. Some researchers in Japan became aware of these risks, although this knowledge was not well disseminated among general practitioners. The intramuscular injections causing muscle contracture were administered by pediatricians, obstetricians, and physicians, whereas the disease was treated by orthopedics. Exchange of information between those conducting the injections and those treating the disease was not close or satisfactory, and this fact was highly likely to bring about the lack of recognition of the risks associated with intramuscular injections. In addition, medical societies and organizations consisting of healthcare professionals such as the Japan Medical Association did not play adequate roles. In 1976, the Japan Pediatric Society issued its proposals as listed below, and requested all relevant medical societies and associations to follow these proposals.

- Give an injection not at a request of a patient's parent but on the basis of medical judgment of the medical doctor.
- Avoid injection as much as possible when treating common cold (syndrome).

裁判で明らかになったこととして，製薬会社による有害事象情報の収集や分析が不十分であり，健康被害の可能性について，医療関係者に的確に情報伝達できていなかったことが指摘されています。さらに製薬会社の責任について，「製薬会社の組織力をもってすれば副作用を掌握することは容易で可能であり，医師に注意，警告を可能な限り伝達する義務を有している」と認定されました。製薬会社の情報収集，分析，対策，伝達義務について明確な司法判断がなされました。

- Avoid injection whenever oral administration is practicable.
- Avoid injecting an antibiotic in combination with other medicines.
- Do not perform subcutaneous injection in large doses.

According to these proposals, injections are currently avoided as much as possible.

The trials revealed that the collection and analyses of information on adverse events by the pharmaceutical companies were inadequate, and that the possibility of intramuscular injection-induced health damage was not adequately communicated to the healthcare professionals. The courts recognized the liability of the pharmaceutical companies by adjudicating as follows: "The pharmaceutical companies have sufficient organizational strength to easily capture and identify occurrences of adverse drug reactions, and also have the duty to communicate relevant notices and warnings as much as possible to medical doctors". The judicial decision was clearly and definitely made on the duties for the pharmaceutical companies to collect, analyze, and deliver the relevant information as well as to take any responsive action relating to the information, if necessary.

7 ダイアライザーによる眼障害事件

事件の概要

　1982年に大阪を中心とする地区のいくつかの病院で，人工透析患者に原因不明の結膜炎様の症状が多発し，眼球の充血，頭痛，吐き気などが厚生省に報告されました。大阪府が直ちに調査を行った結果，患者数は60人を超え，ダイアライザーに原因があることが判明しました。

　厚生省が国立衛生試験所に原因究明を依頼した結果，原料や製造工程，製造管理の不備による不純物の混入，さらに原料中の不純物に起因するという複合的な原因であることがわかりました。まず，製造工程管理の問題として，接着剤として使用されたウレタン樹脂の重合工程管理が不良であったために，生成した低分子重合物質が血液中に溶出したことが原因の一つでした。

　第2に，品質管理の不備から不良品が出荷されていました。品質試験の規格も試験の実施も不適切なため，不良品が出荷検査を通過していました。

　第3の問題は，ホローファイバーに詰められていたグリセリンに含まれていた不純物にありました。使用されたグリセリンは日本薬局方に適合するものでしたが，食用油の廃油を原料に製造されており，その廃油には食品添加物である抗酸化剤が含まれていました。この抗酸化剤が血液中に直接入って，健康被害を起こしました。

　第4の問題として，健康被害の発生が一部の医療機関に偏っていたことから，ダイアライザーの使用方法に問題があることが判明しました。ダイアライザーは生理食塩水で洗浄して使用する器具ですが，これらの医療現場ではコストや時間の節約が優先されていたことから，ダイアライザーの生理食塩水での洗浄が不十分であったとされています。

7 | Dialyzer Induced Ophthalmologic Disorders Incident

Summary of the incident

In 1982, conjunctivitis-like symptoms of unknown causes frequently developed in patients undergoing dialysis treatment at several hospitals in some districts of Osaka and surrounding cities, and the occurrences of bulbar hyperemia, headache, nausea, and other events were reported to the Ministry of Health and Welfare. The Osaka Prefectural Government immediately conducted a survey, which revealed that more than 60 patients suffered from these ophthalmologic disorders and that dialyzers was the cause.

At the request of the Ministry of Health and Welfare, the National Institute of Hygienic Sciences tried to identify the cause of the disorders, and found multiple causes as follows: (1) ingress of impurities due to inadequate control of raw materials and manufacturing processes as well as incomplete manufacturing management; and (2) impurities contained in the raw materials themselves. One of the causes was related to inadequate control of manufacturing processes; polymerization process of urethane resin used as an adhesive was inadequately controlled, causing the formed low molecular weight polymer to dissolve in blood.

The second cause was related to inadequate quality control, leading to shipment of defective products. The specifications for quality tests and the tests themselves were not adequate, allowing defective products to pass shipment inspections.

The third cause was the existence of impurities contained in glycerin which filled the hollow fibers of the device. The glycerin used met the requirements prescribed by the Japanese Pharmacopoeia, but was made from waste cooking oil, which contained an antioxidant as a food additive. The antioxidant directly entered the bloodstream, causing the health damage.

The fourth cause was related to the use of dialyzers since the adverse effects occurred only in some medical institutions, where it was revealed that costs and time saving were given priority and dialyzers were not thoroughly washed with physiological saline, although this washing should be done before use.

ダイアライザー事件に学ぶ

　医薬品の製造については1980年にGMPが法制化されましたが，医療機器にはまだ規制がありませんでした。事件当時，ダイアライザーの価格は保険制度の中で統一価格であり，300〜400億円規模の市場に約30社が競合していたという状況でした。そのため，製造工程や品質管理などが不十分であったことが事件の背景にありました。事件を契機として，医療機器の製造についてもGMPが導入されました。

　日本薬局方では，通常想定される製造方法に対する規格が定められています。しかし，食用油の廃油を原料に使う製造方法は想定されていませんでした。このため，抗酸化剤を含んでいても最終製品は規格試験をすり抜けたのです。この事例は，薬局方の規格に限界があることを示したものと言えます。このため現在は，日本薬局方の規格は合格基準（十分条件）ではなく，個々の製品の製造方法に応じた追加規格試験が必要という考え方になっています。2002年の薬事法改正により，製造方法を承認書に詳しく記載することとなりました。製造方法と品質規格は一体であるべきという考え方です。

　この事件は原因究明が迅速であったこと，大阪府の行政機関が早期の回収措置を講じたことから，被害の拡大を防ぐことができました。これにより，企業と被害者の和解も早期に成立して事件は終息しました。行政と企業の的確な対応が，いかに重要であるかを示した事例です。

Lessons learned from the dialyzer induced ophthalmologic disorders incident

The Good Manufacturing Practice (GMP) for manufacture of drugs was formally legalized as a Ministerial Ordinance in 1980, whereas no such regulations were formulated for medical devices. When the dialyzer-induced suffering occurred, the unified price was applied to dialyzers under the National Health Insurance scheme, at which time about 30 companies were competitive in the dialyzer market corresponding to the size of 30 to 40 billion yen. Under these circumstances, manufacturing processes and quality control were not adequately performed. These background situations had something to do with the development of the suffering that resulted. The dialyzer-induced suffering facilitated introduction of GMP for manufacture of medical devices.

The Japanese Pharmacopoeia defines the specifications for typically expected manufacturing methods. Since the use of waste cooking oil as raw materials to manufacture glycerin was not expected, the responsible dialyzer slipped through the specifications and testing methods for the final product even though it contained the antioxidant. This incident demonstrates the limitations of the specifications of Pharmacopoeias. It is therefore considered that the specifications defined by the Japanese Pharmacopoeia do not represent criteria for acceptance (sufficient conditions) but require additional specifications and testing methods appropriate for manufacturing methods of individual products. The 2002 amendment of the Pharmaceutical Affairs Law makes it mandatory to detail the manufacturing methods as much as possible in the approval form, on the basis of the policy that the manufacturing methods should be integrated with the quality specifications.

Expansion of the dialyzer-induced suffering was avoided firstly because the causes were promptly identified and secondly because the administrative agency of Osaka Prefectural Government immediately ordered recall of the products concerned. A settlement between the responsible companies and the victims was reached promptly and this incident quickly came to an end, which highlights the importance of adequate responsive actions taken by the government and the companies concerned.

8 エイズ事件

事件の概要

　エイズ事件は，サリドマイド事件と同様に世界的な広がりを持った薬害でした。HIV（Human Immunodeficiency Virus）に汚染された原料血漿と血漿分画製剤が，アメリカから輸入されたことによります。しかしその経緯は，日本独自の状況が絡んでいます。

　1964年に発生したライシャワー事件を契機として，日本では1974年頃に，輸血用血液は全量を国内の献血で賄う体制になっていました。一方，血友病患者の治療には輸血と血漿輸注が行われていました。その後，血漿分画部分から血液凝固因子を取りだした製剤，すなわちクリオ製剤が開発されました。その後，2,000人から2万人の血液を集めて，血液凝固因子を抽出して製造した「濃縮血液凝固因子製剤」（濃縮製剤）が使用されるようになりました。1975年頃の日本は，アルブミン製剤などを含めて世界の血漿製剤総量の三分の一を消費していました。したがって，血友病患者の治療にも米国から大量の濃縮製剤を輸入していました。一方で，治療効果の低いクリオ製剤は国内の献血を原料として製造されていました。しかし治療効果の高い濃縮製剤の自己注射が健康保険で認められたこともあって（1978年），血友病治療に濃縮製剤を使用する需要は大きくなっていました。当時の濃縮血液凝固因子製剤は非加熱製剤でした。

　1981年ころから，米国でエイズという奇病が発生しはじめ，エイズ患者の中に血友病患者が高い比率で含まれているという情報から，米国では非加熱濃縮製剤の安全性に懸念がもたれるようになりました。しかし当時日本では，エイズ患者の発生はないとされ，その危険性も評価できない状況でした。このため厚生省は1983年にエイズ研究班（エイズの実態把握に関する研究班）を組織し，エイズ患者の存在確認から始まりました。その研究班の班長には血友病治療の権威者として知られていた専門家が指名されました。班長は当初，非加熱濃縮製剤の全面使用禁止を主張していましたが，なぜかその後に非加熱濃縮製剤の使用継続を決めました。

　1982～1986年に米国から輸入された非加熱濃縮製剤はHIVに汚染されていました。日本には約5,000人の血友病患者がいましたが，うち2,000人近くがこの汚染された非加熱濃縮製剤によってHIVに感染，エイズを発症して死亡するという事態に発展しました。日本でエイズと輸入非加熱濃縮製剤の危険性が認識され，HIV対策としての加熱濃縮製剤が

8 AIDS Incident

Summary of the incident

Like the thalidomide tragedy, the acquired immunodeficiency syndrome (AIDS) incident was of a worldwide scale. The root cause of the incident in Japan was the import of source plasma and plasma derivatives tainted with human immunodeficiency virus (HIV) from the US. How the incident developed and progressed was unique to Japan.

In Japan, a 100% voluntary blood donation system was established in 1974 after the then American Ambassador to Japan, Edwin O. Reischauer, became infected with serum hepatitis as a result of a tainted blood transfusion he received in 1964. Blood transfusions and plasma infusions were performed to treat hemophilia. Subsequently, cryoprecipitate preparations, which were prepared by taking out blood coagulation factors from plasma derivatives, were developed. Following this, "blood coagulation factor concentrate products" (concentrate products), which were prepared by extracting blood coagulation factors from pooled blood collected from 2,000 to 20,000 people, became commercially available. In around 1975, Japan consumed approximately one-third of the total world plasma preparations, including albumin preparations, and imported large quantities of concentrate products from the US for the treatment of hemophilia. On the other hand, cryoprecipitate preparations were manufactured from donated blood in Japan but these drugs provided only low-level effectiveness. Since self-injection of the concentrate products highly effective for the treatment of hemophilia became covered by the Japanese National Health Insurance scheme (in 1978), patients with hemophilia increasingly demanded the concentrate products. The blood coagulation factor concentrate products commercially available at that time were non-heat-treated ones.

In the US, a mysterious disease named AIDS began to occur in around 1981 and it was estimated that hemophilics accounted for a great proportion of AIDS patients. In the US, this information raised concern about the safety of non-heated concentrate products. However, at that time in Japan, it was considered that there were no patients with AIDS and no one could evaluate even the risk of AIDS. In 1983, the Ministry of Health and Welfare organized an AIDS Advisory Panel (to perform fact-finding survey on AIDS), which first of all had to confirm whether or not there were AIDS patients in Japan. A specialist known as an authority on hemophilia treatment was designated as the head of this panel. He initially insisted on banning the use of all non-heat-treated concentrate

承認されたのは1985年でした。このとき，非加熱濃縮製剤を販売していた企業は回収を直ちに行いませんでした。回収が完了したのは，加熱濃縮製剤の承認から2年9か月後のことでした。この間に新たな感染と死亡者が発生しました。

　エイズ事件は，刑事裁判と民事裁判の両方で訴訟が行われました。日本の薬害史上，製薬企業のトップ，医師，官僚が刑事責任を問われた初めての事件でした。血友病の専門家であり医師であったエイズ研究班の班長は，彼が勤務する病院の診療科における責任者として，血友病患者に非加熱濃縮製剤を投与しHIVに感染させ，エイズを発症させて死亡にいたらせたことを問われました。一審では危険性の予見の程度は低かったとして無罪となりました。検察は高裁に上告しましたが，途中で被告が死亡したため公訴棄却となりました。

　企業のトップは，1985年には安全な加熱濃縮製剤が承認されたにもかかわらず，その後も非加熱製剤を販売し，感染を生じさせたことが問われました。この裁判で企業のトップは，「厚生省が回収命令を出さなかったからだ」と争いました。裁判は最高裁まで争われましたが，2被告は実刑が確定し，1被告は途中死亡のため公訴棄却となりました。

　薬害事件は回収が適切な時期に，確実に行われなかったために被害が拡大しました。加熱濃縮製剤が承認されて国内の供給量が十分になり，一方，非加熱濃縮製剤の危険性が容易に認識される状況になっていたにもかかわらず，厚生省の担当課長は回収命令を出しませんでした。このため，回収されなかった非加熱濃縮製剤を投与された手術患者がエイズを発症して死亡したことから，業務上過失致死を問われました。最高裁は被告の上訴を棄却し有罪が確定しました。このように，本事件では回収命令権限を持つ行政の過失と回収義務を持つ企業の怠慢が一対の構造をなしたと言えます。

products but later, for some unexplained reason, decided to allow continued use of non-heated concentrate products.

Non-heated concentrate products imported from the US between 1982 and 1986 were contaminated with HIV. Of about 5,000 hemophilics who existed in Japan at that time, almost 2,000 became infected with the virus through these HIV tainted concentrate products, contracted AIDS, and died. In Japan, it was not until 1985 that the risk of AIDS development due to the imported non-heated concentrate products was recognized and heat-treated concentrate products were approved as a measure to control HIV infection. At that time, however, the pharmaceutical companies that marketed non-heated concentrate products did not immediately retrieve the products from the market. The retrieval was completed 2 years and 9 months after the approval of heat-treated concentrate products. During this interval, new cases of infection and deaths occurred.

The AIDS incident brought about both criminal and civil lawsuits. In the trials, top management executives of a pharmaceutical company, a medical doctor, and a government official faced criminal charges, the first such Japanese court cases of drug-induced sufferings. The medical doctor, who was a specialist of hemophilia and the head of the AIDS Advisory Panel, was accused of allowing, as a responsible person of the clinic of the hospital he worked for, one of the hemophilics to be treated with non-heated concentrate products, which caused HIV infection, development of AIDS, and eventually death. The district court ruled that he was not criminally responsible for the death because it was judged difficult for him to have foreseen that the event would occur. The prosecution appealed to the high court. However, since the medical doctor died in the mid-course of the appeal trial, the high court dismissed the case.

The top management executives of the pharmaceutical company were accused of continuing to market the non-heated concentrate products even after 1985, by which time a safe, heat-treated concentrate product was approved, resulting in infection with the virus. In the litigation, the executives of the drug firm claimed that the company alone could not decide to recall the product without receiving instructions from the Ministry of Health and Welfare. The case was brought to the Supreme Court. Two of the 3 defendant executives were sentenced to prison terms, and for the third, who died in the mid-course of the appeal trial, the case was dismissed.

In the AIDS incident in Japan, the disaster expanded because the recalls were not conducted in a timely manner and without fail. Specifically, despite the facts that heat-treated concentrate products were approved and their supply was sufficient to meet the needs in Japan, and in addition, that the risks associated with the non-heated concentrate products were easily recognized due to information already available, the responsible Director of the Ministry of Health and Welfare did not order drug

エイズ事件に学ぶ

　当時，日本の医薬品開発は独自のGCPで規定される「治験総括医師」という専門家が開発の方向性，治験組織，実施，さらには承認申請の時期まで影響を与えていました。この専門家が加熱濃縮製剤の開発と承認においても，開発企業間の調整を図ったという問題が指摘されています。これをきっかけとして，ICH-GCPが日本に導入され治験の質の向上と企業責任の明確化が図られました。

　審査段階においては生物由来製品は化学医薬品とは異なると認識されており，審査，国家検定，薬事監視まで一貫して生物製剤課が担当していました。したがって化学医薬品を担当する審査部門，安全性部門や監視部門，感染症部門などとの連携が不十分であったために，欧米における最新の感染症情報，安全性情報，薬事監視情報が活かされず，状況認識に遅れと判断の誤りにつながったとされます。

　市販後の段階では，生物製剤課は生物製剤のすべてを一貫して担当した部署で，いわゆる縦割り組織でした。縦割り組織はうまく機能しているときには効率的ですが，いったん問題が起きると情報の共有がされにくく，問題が拡大しやすい危険があります。このため，厚生行政では生物製剤と化学医薬品という区別を排除した，審査・安全対策・監視組織体制に組織変更が行われました。

　血液製剤は，原料がヒト由来の非常に貴重な製剤でありながら，日本における使用量が非常に多かったことが事件の素地となりました。これはCJD事件と共通する点でした。また血液製剤が適応外にも多く使われたことが需要を増大させ，ひいては被害を拡大させたことにもつながりました。薬事規制とは別の問題が提起されます。

　血液製剤の汚染による感染被害は既存の医薬品副作用被害救済制度の対象とならないことが大きな問題となり，2004年から生物由来製品による感染被害救済制度が導入されました。さらに医療現場では生物由来製品の保管，使用管理，記録などが十分でなかったために問題が発生した時の追跡が十分に行えないことが分かり，一般医薬品に対する要求事項に加えて生物由来という特性を踏まえた上乗せ要求事項が，2002年の薬事法改正で設

firms to recall the non-heated products. He was charged with professional negligence since a patient received a non-heated concentrate product that should not have been available had the defendant ordered the recall, contracted AIDS, and died. The Supreme Court dismissed an appeal by the defendant and he was found guilty. The AIDS incident was caused by a combination of negligence of the government, which had the authority to order recalls, and negligence of drug firms, which had a duty to recall products.

Lessons learned from the AIDS incident

In the 1980s, when the AIDS incident occurred in Japan, the expert called "principal investigator" that was defined by Japan's unique GCP had influence on the direction of development, organization involved in clinical trials, and conduct of clinical trials, and even the timing of when to submit applications for approval of drug products. This gave rise to a problem that such experts intentionally regulated the progress of development and even approval-related activities for heat-treated concentrate products among the pharmaceutical companies engaged in the development. This incident facilitated the introduction of ICH-GCP in Japan with the aim of improving the quality of clinical trials and defining the responsibilities of pharmaceutical companies.

Biological products were considered different from synthesized drugs at the stage of reviews of applications for new drugs and accordingly, the Biologics Division, Ministry of Health and Welfare took responsibilities for all aspects relating to reviews for biological products, i.e. reviews of applications for new drugs and, national inspection through to pharmacovigilance. This system resulted in inadequate cooperation with functions responsible for synthesized drugs with regards to drug reviews for approval, safety measures and pharmacovigilance, infection control, and other relevant duties. As a result of this inadequate collaboration, the latest information on infections, safety, and pharmacovigilance that was obtained in European and North American countries was not effectively utilized, leading to delayed identification of what was going on and eventually, resulted in the wrong decisions.

The Biologics Division took all responsibilities relating to biological products, including those in the post-marketing phase. This was a vertically split organization. Such sectionalism is efficient when all is going well, but when a problem occurs, it can be difficult for information to be shared with other relevant functions, which may escalate or mask the problem. For this reason the organization for drug administration was changed; functions responsible for drug review for approval, safety measures, and pharmacovigilance exist without having the distinction between biological products and synthesized drugs.

定されました。

　生物由来製品は常に未知の微生物に汚染の危険の可能性がありますが，患者への説明，告知などが十分に行われていない実態が明らかになりました。この汚染の危険性について感染症定期報告制度が導入されました。これは，最新の論文などにより得られた知見に基づいた評価を，厚生労働大臣に定期的に報告するものです。

　このようにエイズ事件はサリドマイド事件以来の薬事規制の不足，不備を明らかにしたと言えます。

Raw materials of blood products are derived from humans and thus are extremely valuable. Japan's consumption of valuable plasma source was extremely large, which formed the foundation for the development of the AIDS incident. This feature, i.e. Japan's prominent consumption of raw materials of human origin, was also noted in the case of prion infection caused by human dura mater grafts (i.e. the Creutzfeldt-Jakob Disease (CJD) incident). In Japan, the blood products were frequently used in a way not specified in the labeling approved by the regulatory authorities (i.e. "off-label-use"), which increased the demand of blood products and eventually expanded the disaster. These facts raise issues unrelated to the pharmaceutical regulatory system.

The existing Relief System for Adverse Drug Reactions was not applied to the infections acquired through contaminated blood products and this became a major issue. In 2004, the Relief System for Infections Acquired through Biological Products was established. Furthermore, it was revealed that since storage, management of use, and keeping necessary records for biological products were not adequate in clinical settings, and thus traceability was not properly achieved when a problem occurred. The amendment of the Pharmaceutical Affairs Law in 2002 set new requirements based on the characteristics of biological products, in addition to the existing requirements specified for pharmaceutical products.

It was also identified that patients were not given clear and adequate explanation of the risks of contamination associated with biological products, although biologics may always be at risk of being contaminated with unknown microorganisms. For handling the risks of contamination, the system of periodic reporting of infections was introduced, according to which manufacturers of biological products must evaluate their products based on findings obtained from the latest relevant papers or articles and periodically report the evaluation results to the Minister of Health, Labour and Welfare.

As described above, the AIDS incident identified weaknesses and imperfections of the pharmaceutical regulatory system that persisted following the thalidomide incident.

9 血液製剤（フィブリノゲン）によるHCV感染事件

事件の概要

　C型肝炎感染事件は，エイズ事件と同じく第VIII因子製剤，第IX因子製剤によるものの他，フィブリノゲン製剤によっても引き起こされました。ここでは，感染の主体となったフィブリノゲン製剤について概要を記述します。エイズ事件は米国から輸入された原料血漿等がHIVに汚染されていたことが原因でしたが，C型肝炎事件も米国から輸入された原料血漿がHCVに汚染されていたことが原因でした。エイズ事件と異なるのは，フィブリノゲン製剤が産科も含め多くの診療科でも広く使われたことです。

　日本でフィブリノゲンが承認されたのは1964年でした。当時，輸血や血液製剤の使用による肝炎の発生は比較的少ないものでした。しかし1972年，厚生省は難治性の肝炎研究班を設置し，非A非B型肝炎，すなわちC型肝炎の存在について調査研究を行い，その存在が示唆されました。

　1975年に出血性ショックによる妊婦死亡の措置をめぐる裁判で，東京地裁は「大量出血時にフィブリノゲン製剤を投与するなど適切な措置を取らなかった」として，産科医師に高額の賠償を命じました。このことが出産時の出血や外傷，手術時の止血にフィブリノゲン製剤が多用されることに拍車をかけることとなりました。

　一方，米国では1977年12月に，FDAがフィブリノゲン製剤のB型肝炎ウイルス汚染の危険性及び臨床効果が疑わしいとして，その承認を取り消しました。日本では1978年2月，当該の製薬企業では，米国での承認取り消しの情報が社内で回覧されていました。さらに1979年には，国立予防衛生研究所血液製剤部長が自著の中で米国での承認取り消しに言及しましたが，この情報は厚生省には伝わっていませんでした。

　1985年，当該企業は厚生省に製造方法の一部変更申請を行わないまま，無断でウイルス不活性化法をBPL処理（β-プロピオラクトン酸の添加）から抗HBsグロブリン添加法に変更しました。実はBPL処理法でHCVは不活化されていたのですが，変更後は不活化が不十分であったために，HCV汚染が拡大することになりました。

　C型感染が社会問題化したのは1987年，青森県の産婦人科医院で非加熱フィブリノゲ

9 | Blood Product (Fibrinogen) Induced HCV Infection Incident

Summary of the incident

Drug-induced infection with Hepatitis C virus (HCV) was caused by coagulation factor VIII and IX products, as in the AIDS incident, and in addition, by fibrinogen products. In this section, the HCV infection incident is summarized by focusing on fibrinogen products that played a major role in HCV infection. The AIDS incident was caused by HIV-tainted source plasma and plasma derivatives imported from the US. The HCV infection incident was again caused by HCV-tainted source plasma imported from the US, although the difference from the AIDS incident was that fibrinogen products were widely used in various clinics including departments of obstetrics.

In Japan, a fibrinogen product was officially approved in 1964. At that time, hepatitis was caused only infrequently by blood transfusion or use of blood products. In 1972, the Ministry of Health and Welfare (MHW) organized an advisory panel for refractory hepatitis to perform a survey and research on non-A, non-B type hepatitis, i.e. hepatitis C, and the presence of hepatitis C was suggested.

In 1975, for a lawsuit regarding the issue of adequacy of treatment for a pregnant woman who died of hemorrhage shock, the Tokyo District Court ordered the defendant obstetrician to pay substantial financial compensation by adjudicating as follows: "The obstetrician did not take an appropriate action, such as administration of fibrinogen products, when massive hemorrhage occurred". This ruling accelerated frequent use of fibrinogen products to control hemorrhage during childbirth, upon treatment of injuries, and during surgery.

In the US, the Food and Drug Administration (FDA) withdrew its approval of the fibrinogen products in December 1977 since they identified risks of hepatitis B viral contamination of the products and raised doubts regarding their clinical efficacy. In February 1978 in Japan, the pharmaceutical company concerned distributed inside the company information about the US withdrawal. Furthermore, in 1979, a person who was the Director of the Blood Products Division, National Institute of Health in Japan mentioned in his own book that the US government withdrew the approval of the fibrinogen products, although this information was not communicated to the MHW.

ン製剤を投与された産婦8人が，C型肝炎に集団感染したことが新聞報道されたことによります。厚生省は当該企業に調査報告を求め，74人の感染が報告されました。同時に企業は，非加熱の血液製剤を自主回収し，製剤すべてを破棄しました。その直後に加熱フィブリノゲン製剤が製造承認されました。しかし自主回収は徹底せず，1988年に厚生省の指示により非加熱製剤についての緊急安全性情報が発出され，医療機関に返品を求めました。

1990年に加熱製剤が再評価指定となり，臨床的有用性の検討が始まりましたが，1997年に企業が後天性低フィブリノゲン血症に対する有用性の試験を断念し，1998年に厚生省はその適応症を，先天性無または低フィブリノゲン血症に限定しました。

HCV感染事件に学ぶ

本事件に関しては，厚生労働省が2002年に「フィブリノゲン製剤によるC型肝炎ウイルス感染に関する調査報告書」を取りまとめました。これを受けて以下の対応がなされました。

・当該企業が一部変更承認申請を行わず，また肝炎調査の結果を厚生省に過小報告していたとみられたことから，2002年の薬事法改正では企業の責任を明確にしました。つまり，医薬品等の市場への供給を行うものを新たに「製造販売業者」と位置付け，製品に対する企業責任を明確化するとともに，製造販売業者の許可要件に市販後安全要件が追加されました。さらに，危害発生時における製品の廃棄，回収，販売停止，情報提供の措置に関する企業の責務が法律的に明確化されました。

In 1985, the pharmaceutical company concerned changed the viral inactivation method from BPL treatment (addition of β-propiolactone) to addition of anti-HBs globulin, without making an application for approval for partial change in the approved manufacturing methods to the MHW. In fact, the BPL treatment method had inactivated the HCV, whereas after the change, viral inactivation was inadequate, resulting in expansion of HCV contamination.

In 1987, an outbreak of hepatitis C infection in an obstetrics clinic occurred in Aomori Prefecture. Eight pregnant women given the non-heated fibrinogen product all contracted the virus, which was reported in the newspapers, and made hepatitis C infection a social issue. The NHW requested the responsible company to conduct a survey, and the survey identified 74 such cases that were reported to the MHW. At the same time, this company voluntarily retrieved the non-heated blood product from the market and destroyed all of the retrieved drugs. Immediately after, the same company obtained an official approval for manufacture of a heat-treated fibrinogen product. However, the voluntary recall was not thoroughly performed. In 1988, the company issued an Urgent Safety Information about the non-heated product in response to the order given by the Ministry of Health and Welfare, and requested all medical institutions to return the product to the company.

In 1990, the heat-treated fibrinogen product was designated by the regulatory authorities as a drug subject to reevaluation, and investigation of its clinical usefulness was begun. In 1997, the company concerned abandoned studies for evaluation of its usefulness in the treatment of acquired hypofibrinogenemia. In 1998, the MHW limited the indication of this heat-treated fibrinogen product to congenital afibrinogenemia and congenital hypofibrinogenemia.

Lessons learned from the blood product (fibrinogen) induced HCV infection incident

For this incident, the Ministry of Health, Labour and Welfare prepared the "Report of Survey on Infection with Hepatitis C Virus Acquired through Fibrinogen Preparation" in 2002, on the basis of which the actions listed below were taken.

- The responsible company did not make an application for approval for partial change in the approved manufacturing methods to the regulatory authorities, and in addition, reported to the Ministry of Health and Welfare a smaller number of cases of hepatitis than that actually revealed by the survey they conducted. Given these facts, the amendment of the Pharmaceutical Affairs Law in 2002 clarified the responsibilities of companies. More specifically, the amendment prescribed as follows: the person who starts supply of drugs, etc. to the market is defined as the

・2002年の薬事法改正では，薬局，病院等の医療関係者を対象に副作用等症例の厚生労働大臣への報告規定を創設しました。これにより，企業による情報収集と報告が十分に履行されない場合の補完体制が整備されました。

・エイズ事件でも同様のことが生じましたが，国立感染症研究所の把握していた情報が十分に活用されなかったことから1997年，厚生省は健康危機管理基本方針と医薬品等健康危機管理実施要領を制定しました。

・エイズ事件，薬害肝炎事件を契機として2002年に「採血及び供血あっせん業取締法」を「安全な血液製剤の安定供給の確保等に関する法律」として抜本的に改訂しました。

　厚生労働省が取りまとめた報告書とは別に，薬害肝炎の全国原告団，全国弁護団と厚生労働省との合意に基づく委員会が設立されました。この委員会は，①薬害肝炎事件の検証と，②再発防止のための医薬品行政の在り方の検討，という二つの役割を担って2010年に最終報告書を取りまとめました（第4章参照）。

　フィブリノゲン製剤は止血剤として，産科以外でも多用されました。しかし再評価で，その適応は極めて限られることとなりました。裏返せば，エビデンスのないままに広く使われてしまったことが，C型肝炎を日本に蔓延させてしまったと言えます。この事例で取り上げたフィブリノゲン製剤は，6,000の医療機関に納入されて30万人に投与され，1万人が感染したと言われていますが，その他の感染を含めると感染者350万人という推定もあります。血液製剤の多くが止血目的に使われました。同時に患者は輸血を受けていることが多く，C型肝炎の感染経路が血液製剤によるものなのか，輸血によるものなのか不明な場合が多いとされています。国は2009年に肝炎対策基本法を成立させ，C型肝炎患者の救済を行うことになりました。

"marketing authorization holder (MAH)"; the responsibilities of the MAH for the products marketed are clarified; the requirements for a MAH to obtain a license are expanded to include additional ones regarding post-marketing safety; and the legal responsibilities for the responsible companies to destroy, recall, discontinue marketing of, and provide information on a product in case of harm associated with the product are clarified.

- The 2002 amendment of the Pharmaceutical Affairs Law formulated new provisions according to which healthcare professionals at pharmacies, hospitals, etc. must report cases of adverse drug reactions, etc. to the Minister of Health, Labour and Welfare. This reporting system ensures the complete collection of information on adverse drug reactions even if the pharmaceutical companies fail to perform adequate collection and reporting of such information.
- Since the information that the National Institute of Infectious Diseases had possessed was not effectively utilized in this incident (note that the same failure to share relevant information among the stakeholders was identified in the AIDS incident), the MHW formulated the "Basic Policy for Health Risk Management" and the "Implementation Guidance for Health Risk Management on Drugs. Etc." in 1997.
- The AIDS incident and the drug-induced hepatitis incident resulted in a drastic reform of the "Blood Collection and Donation Service Control Law" so as to enact the "Law on Securing Stable Supply of Safe Blood Products" in 2002.

In addition to the report prepared by the Ministry of Health, Labour and Welfare, a committee was organized on the basis of the agreement reached by the nationwide plaintiffs' group, the nationwide defendants' group, and the Ministry of Health, Labour and Welfare. This committee had two duties, i.e. (1) to verify the drug-induced hepatitis, and (2) to explore the desirable drug administration for prevention of its recurrence, and published its final report in 2010 (See Chapter 4).

Fibrinogen products were frequently used as hemostatic therapy in various departments other than those of obstetrics. The reevaluation of these products extremely narrowed their indications. When looking at these facts from the opposite direction, we can say that the widespread use of fibrinogen products without evidence allowed hepatitis C to sweep across Japan. The fibrinogen product involved in the incident described here was delivered to 6,000 medical institutions and administered to 300,000 patients, of whom 10,000 contracted the virus. Another estimation indicates that the number of individuals infected with hepatitis viruses totals as high as 3.5 million. Although blood products are primarily administered to control hemorrhage, it is unknown in many cases if hepatitis C infection is caused by blood products or blood transfusion since those given blood products frequently receive blood transfusion concomitantly. The Japanese government established the "Basic Act on Hepatitis Measures" in 2009 for the purpose of providing relief benefits to patients with hepatitis C.

肝炎対策基本法の立法趣旨

　今日，わが国には，肝炎ウイルスに感染し，あるいは肝炎に罹患した者が多数存在し，肝炎が国内最大の感染症となっている。肝炎は，適切な治療を行わないまま放置すると慢性化し，肝硬変，肝がんといったより重篤な疾病に進行するおそれがあることから，これらの者にとって，将来への不安は計り知れないものがある。

　戦後の医療の進歩，医学的知見の積重ね，科学技術の進展により，肝炎の克服に向けた道筋が開かれてきたが，他方で，現在においても，早期発見や医療へのアクセスにはいまだ解決すべき課題が多く，さらには，肝炎ウイルスや肝炎に対する正しい理解が，国民すべてに定着しているとは言えない。

　B型肝炎及びC型肝炎に係るウイルスへの感染については，国の責めに帰すべき事由によりもたらされ，又はその原因が解明されていなかったことによりもたらされたものがある。特定の血液凝固因子製剤にC型肝炎ウイルスが混入することによって不特定多数の者に感染被害を出した薬害肝炎事件では，感染被害者の方々に甚大な被害が生じ，その被害の拡大を防止し得なかったことについて国が責任を認め，集団予防接種の際の注射器の連続使用によってB型肝炎ウイルスの感染被害を出した予防接種禍事件では，最終の司法判断において国の責任が確定している。

　このような現状において，肝炎ウイルスの感染者及び肝炎患者の人権を尊重しつつ，これらの者に対する良質かつ適切な医療の提供を確保するなど，肝炎の克服に向けた取組を一層進めていくことが求められている。ここに，肝炎対策に係る施策について，その基本理念を明らかにするとともに，これを総合的に推進するためこの法律を制定する。

Purposes of Establishing the "Basic Act on Hepatitis Measures"

Today, many people in Japan are infected with hepatitis viruses or have contracted hepatitis. Hepatitis is the most widespread infectious disease in Japan. Those infected with the virus or the infection have incalculable anxiety about the future since hepatitis can become chronic and progress into more severe diseases such as cirrhosis or liver cancer if left without proper treatment.

The path to conquer hepatitis has been opened, thanks to the advancement of medical care, accumulation of medical knowledge, and development of science and technology in the post-war period, although there are still many challenges to overcome in terms of early detection and accessibility of medical care. Furthermore, it cannot be said that all Japanese citizens have an accurate understanding of hepatitis virus and hepatitis.

Infection with hepatitis B and C viruses was in some cases caused by factors the national government should be responsible for, and in other cases induced by the fact that the causes of acquisition of the infection were unknown. In the case of drug-induced hepatitis C, particular blood coagulation factor products tainted with hepatitis C virus caused an unspecified large number of people to contract the virus, and the victims with infection suffered serious harm. The national government admitted its responsibility and liability for failing to prevent the spread of such harm. In the case of vaccination-induced suffering, in which the reuse of syringes and needles upon mass vaccination caused infection with hepatitis B virus, the national government's liability has been settled by final judicial decision.

Under these circumstances, further and greater commitment is required to take actions so as to overcome hepatitis, e.g. by securing high-quality and appropriate medical care for carriers of hepatitis virus and hepatitis patients, whilst still respecting their human rights. The "Basic Act on Hepatitis Measures" was established to clarify the basic principles of the hepatitis measures and to comprehensively promote those measures.

10 陣痛促進剤事件

事件の概要

　現在の日本では99％の新生児が病院で誕生しています。日本において，出産が助産婦の助けを借りて家庭や助産所で行われる状況から病院で出産する傾向が強くなったのは，1970年代の後半からでした。このころから陣痛促進剤の使用に関連して，子宮破裂，頸管裂傷，弛緩出血，胎児死亡，新生児仮死に続く脳性まひなどの事故が報告されるようになりました。

　これらの事故の直接の原因は陣痛促進剤の不適切な使用でしたが，その背景には，病院における計画分娩があるとされています。新生児の時間別出生数を見ると，病院の場合では午後2時台にピークがあり，夜間の出産数の倍になっています。しかし助産所の場合では，朝の6時にやや増えて，夕方の6時にやや減るというごく緩やかな変化を示しており，病院とはその傾向が全く違っています。本来，陣痛促進剤は母体や胎児にトラブルが予測されたり，ハイリスク出産の場合に使われるべきものですが，このデータはむしろ，病院の管理の都合が優先されていることを推測させるものです。

　陣痛促進剤の危険性は，薬剤感受性の個人差が非常に大きく，同じ用量でも過強陣痛を生じる場合があることです。1974年に現在の日本産婦人科医会が日本の産科医師に配布した陣痛促進剤に関する小冊子では，陣痛促進剤による事故の頻発とともに，感受性の個人差が200倍以上である，として自動点滴装置を使った注入を指示しています。この冊子は1974年から毎年，全国の産婦人科医に配布されていましたが，陣痛促進剤による被害は減少しませんでした。

　1992年になって，厚生省はようやく添付文書改訂に踏み切りました。しかしその後も事故は続き，2005年には添付文書改訂以降に陣痛促進剤の不適切使用で母子127人が死亡したことが報道されました。2009年から産科医療補償制度が設けられました。この制度は先天性・遺伝子疾患を除き，分娩によって重度の脳性まひになった新生児に対する補償と原因分析，再発防止を目的としたものです。この制度が適用となった最初の15例のうち6例で，陣痛促進剤の添付文書からの大きな逸脱が見られています。厚生科学研究の報告では，出産時に母親が死亡した2005年の197例について，陣痛促進剤が有意に関連していたと結論しています。

10 Labor-Inducing Drugs Incident

Summary of the incident

In Japan, 99% of babies are currently born in hospitals. In contract, in the past, women gave birth with the assistance of midwives at their own home or in midwifery homes. In the latter half of the 1970s, increasing numbers of deliveries were made in hospitals and along with this trend, accidents related to administration of labor-inducing drugs were reported, including, among others, uterine rupture, cervical laceration, atonic hemorrhage, fetal death, and neonatal asphyxia followed by cerebral palsy.

The direct cause of these accidents was improper use of labor-inducing drugs. It is pointed out that planned deliveries at hospitals bring about the improper use of these drugs. Evaluation of the number of newborn babies by time reveals that at hospitals, there is a peak in number of deliveries between 2 and 3 p.m., which is double the number during the night-time. On the other hand, the same parameter at midwifery homes shows a gentle curve with a slight increase at around 6 a.m. and a slight decrease at around 6 p.m., which is totally different from the pattern observed in hospitals. Labor-inducing drugs should only be used when it is expected that a mother or the fetus may experience any trouble or when a delivery may be at high risk. The above-stated data may serve to indicate that hospitals prioritize convenience from the viewpoint of management, rather than focusing on what is best for the mothers and their fetuses.

Labor-inducing drugs are hazardous since drug sensitivity to these agents substantially varies depending on individuals. Even at the same dose, some mothers suffer from excessively strong pains during childbirth, while others do not. In 1974, a booklet on labor-inducing drugs was distributed to Japanese obstetricians by the currently named Japan Association of Obstetricians and Gynecologists. This booklet warned that the use of labor-inducing drugs frequently caused accidents and that the sensitivity to these drugs varied greatly depending on individuals, producing differences by a factor of more than 200 times, and instructed that these drugs must be infused with automatic drip-infusion devices. The booklet was distributed to obstetricians throughout Japan every year starting from 1974, although health damage caused by labor-inducing drugs did not decline.

2010年に再度，添付文書が改定され，陣痛促進剤を用いる必要性とその危険性について，説明と同意を必要とすることが警告事項として追加されました。これにより，陣痛促進剤が妊婦に無断で，もしくは十分な説明なしで使われるということが許されなくなりました。

陣痛促進剤事件に学ぶ

　陣痛促進剤による被害が問題となり始めた1970年代の終わりごろの医師の意識は，今日とは大きく異なります。当時，「医師は医療のプロフェッショナルであり，添付文書に使い方や対処の方法をこと細かく書くことは医師の裁量を侵すものである」という風潮がありました。このため，陣痛促進剤の投与速度などの細かいことは，現場の医師に任されていました。現在では陣痛促進剤の使い方，投与速度，危険性について，添付文書に詳細に書かれています。現在のように，適正使用という概念に基づいて必要な情報を医療関係者に円滑に提供できるまでには，薬害事件を契機とした行政による医療関係者に対する説得の長い道のりが必要でした。陣痛促進剤事件はその典型的な事例の一つです。

　陣痛促進剤事件は，被害者救済に新しいシステムを誕生させました。それが産科医療補償制度です。これは医薬品副作用救済制度とは別の救済システムです。医薬品副作用救済制度による救済金は，裁判での賠償金とは独立しています。一方，産科医療補償制度での救済を受けた場合，金額や条件によっては裁判で得た賠償金額との調整が行われます。また，このシステムによって再発防止を目的として第三者による原因分析を行い，その結果は分娩を行った医療機関にフィードバックするとともに，必要であれば行政や学会などへ報告書を提供しています。この制度は2009年に始まったばかりですが，産科医療の質と信頼の向上にどのように寄与するかが注目されます。

In 1992, the Ministry of Health and Welfare eventually embarked on the revision of package inserts, but accidents continued to occur. In 2005, it was reported by the mass media that despite the revision of package inserts, 127 mothers and their babies had died due to improper use of labor-inducing agents since the revision. In 2009, the Japan Obstetric Compensation System for Cerebral Palsy was established with the aims of providing monetary compensation for babies with severe cerebral palsy related to brain injuries during childbirth, analyzing the causes of accidents, and preventing further similar accidents, although congenital diseases and genetic disorders are not covered by this system. In 6 of the first 15 cases to which this system was applied, substantial deviations from the statements in the package inserts were confirmed. A study officially approved by the Ministry of Health and Welfare under the scheme of Health Science Research concluded that 197 mother deaths upon childbirth in 2005 were significantly related to labor-inducing agents.

In 2010, the package inserts were again revised and the following warning was added: Give thorough explanation to pregnant women of the necessity of using labor-inducing agents and the associated risks, and obtain prior informed consent. This does not allow the use of labor-inducing drugs without obtaining consent from pregnant women or without providing a sufficient explanation.

Lessons learned from the labor-inducing drugs incident

In the closing years of the 1970s, during which sufferings caused by labor-inducing drugs attracted people's attention as a significant issue, the prevailing attitudes and over-confidence of medical doctors were greatly different from those today. At that time, there was a public perception that "medical doctors were professionals in medical care and to describe detailed instructions on how to use a drug and how to take responsive actions in case there were adverse events, if any, in the package insert undermined the doctor's credibility". Under this general mood of the people, the dosing rate or any other detailed matters relating to administration of labor-inducing agents were left to medical doctors. At present, how to use labor-inducing agents, dosing rates, and associated risks are described in detail in the package inserts. Nowadays, on the basis of the concept of the proper use of drugs, necessary information is adequately and effectively provided to healthcare professionals, at which we have finally arrived after struggling to walk a long road of getting healthcare professionals to understand the extreme significance of this matter. Drug-induced sufferings contributed to raising their awareness, and the labor-inducing drugs incident is one such representative event contributing to the establishment of the current drug administration.

The labor-inducing drugs incident gave rise to a new system of providing relief services to victims, i.e. the Japan Obstetric Compensation System for Cerebral Palsy (hereinafter referred to as the

Obstetric Compensation System). This is a separate relief system from the Relief System for Adverse Drug Reactions. The relief benefits under the Relief System for Adverse Drug Reactions are independent of the compensatory damages decided by a court in the trial. When a victim receives relief benefits under the Obstetric Compensation System, depending on the monetary amount of and conditions for such relief benefits, adjustment will be made between the amount of such benefits and the compensatory damages decided by a court's decision. Under the Obstetric Compensation System, the causes of accidents are analyzed by a third-party organization for the purpose of preventing recurrence of similar accidents. The analysis results are given as feedback information to the relevant childbirth facilities, and whenever necessary, reports are submitted to the national government, scientific societies or associations, and any other relevant entities. This System started in 2009 and it remains to be seen how it contributes to improvement of both quality of obstetric institutions and people's trust in these institutions.

11 MMRワクチン事件

事件の概要

MMRワクチンとは麻疹（measles），おたふくかぜ（mumps），風疹（rubella）の頭文字をとったもので，これら3種のワクチンが混合されたものです。日本では1948年に予防接種法が制定され，麻疹，風疹は定期接種として努力義務が課せられていました。1988年に厚生省の予防接種委員会が，「早急に現行の麻疹定期接種時にMMRワクチンを接種できるよう積極的に進めるべきである」との意見書をまとめました。

これを受けて，厚生省は1989年4月からMMRワクチン接種を開始しました。そのワクチンに品質上の問題があり，接種された子供たちに発熱，嘔吐，痙攣を伴う無菌性髄膜炎が発生したのです。1989年から1993年の間に接種された183万人のうち，1,754例の無菌性髄膜炎の報告がありました。およそ1,000人に一人の割合です。重症例は死亡し，また重篤な後遺症は麻痺，難聴，てんかん，知的障害などが残りました。

厚生省の指導により問題のあったワクチンは，ワクチンを製造する3社それぞれで一番実績のある疾患ワクチンを採用し，それを混合することで製造されました。3社は，採用されたワクチンの原液をお互い交換して，同じ規格の下に製造したもの（統一株という）を使うことになりました。しかしおたふくかぜのワクチン原液の製造方法に問題があり，無菌性髄膜炎を発症させる原因となったのです。MMRワクチンは1988年に製造承認され，同年末には法定接種への導入が決定しました。しかしこの時すでに，安全性に関する重要な情報があったのです。

このおたふくかぜのワクチン（占部Am-9株）は海外でも使用され，日本の場合より発症例は少ないのですが，カナダでは1987年9月までに（占部Am-9株を用いた）MMRワクチン接種後に3例の無菌性髄膜炎が発生しました。さらに1988年11月までに8例が報告され，カナダでは製造企業が直ちに製造・販売を中止しました。

一方，日本においてもMMRワクチンの製造承認，導入時におたふくかぜワクチンもしくはMMRワクチン接種後に髄膜炎を発現し，ワクチンとの関連性を疑う症例報告が1983年から1989年にかけて13報ありました。おたふくかぜワクチン原液を製造した企業が把握していた健康被害のデータでは，1989年12月の時点で少なくとも19例の髄膜炎の症例

11 MMR Vaccine Incident

Summary of the incident

MMR stands for measles, mumps, and rubella. The MMR vaccine is a mixture of immunization vaccines against the 3 diseases. In Japan, the Preventive Vaccination Law was established in 1948; it designated vaccinations against measles and rubella as periodic ones, and encouraged children to be vaccinated against these diseases, although no legal punishment was imposed on those who did not receive them. In 1988, the Preventive Vaccination Committee, Ministry of Health and Welfare formulated a recommendation that "the national government should proactively take actions to promptly establish a system of providing MMR vaccination at the time that is currently designated for periodic immunization against measles".

In response to the recommendation, the Ministry of Health and Welfare started MMR vaccination in April 1989. The vaccine used at that time had a quality problem and children given the dose suffered from aseptic meningitis with fever, vomiting, and convulsions. Of 1,830,000 children vaccinated between 1989 and 1993, 1,754 cases of aseptic meningitis were reported. This means that the adverse drug reaction developed in approximately one per 1000 children. Those with critical symptoms died and serious sequelae included, among others, paralysis, hearing losses, epilepsy, and mental disability.

Under the directions given by the Ministry of Health and Welfare, the problematic vaccine was a mixture of 3 components, each of which was separately manufactured by a single pharmaceutical company. The most proven vaccine for one of the 3 diseases that was manufactured by one of the 3 companies was adopted and they were combined to produce the MMR vaccine concerned. Each of the 3 companies provided a single bulk liquid for the adopted vaccine, to the other 2 companies, and manufactured a "3-in-1" vaccine by using the 3 bulk liquids under the same specifications (i.e. the unified strain). The manufacturing methods of the bulk liquid for the mumps vaccine had a problem and this was the cause of the aseptic meningitis. Manufacture of the MMR vaccine was approved in 1988 and at the end of 1988, inclusion of this combination vaccine into the legal vaccination scheme was decided. By the time of this decision, however, there had existed important information regarding safety that should not have been underrated.

があり，これらは当時開発されたPCR法により，おたふくかぜの野生株によるものではなく，ワクチン由来のものであることが判明していました．この情報は公表されず，医療関係者にも共有されませんでした．

1989年，前橋市の医師会は，MMRワクチン接種開始の当初から副作用に関するデータ収集を行いました．それはおたふくかぜに自然感染した子供が髄膜炎を発症することがあり，生ワクチンの接種でも自然感染と同じことが起こりうると想定したことにあります．その結果，217人に一人の割合で髄膜炎の発症していました．この結果は厚生省に報告されましたが，上記の情報と同様に公表も共有もされませんでした．これらの状況が積み重なった結果，接種を行った医師も，行政も，親も，MMRワクチンによる髄膜炎を想像していませんでした．そしてMMRワクチンによる二次感染が，1993年に報告されるに至りました．MMRワクチン接種は同年中止になりました．

MMRワクチンによる健康被害に対して，予防接種健康被害救済制度が適用された被害児は1065人になりました．またこれとは別に，国とワクチン製造企業を被告とした裁判が起されました．地方裁判所での判決は「メーカーは製造方法を無断で変更したこと，国はメーカーが薬事法順守するよう指導する義務があった」として賠償責任を認めました．

The mumps vaccine strain used in the problematic product in Japan was the Urabe Am-9 strain and this strain was also used outside Japan, although the number of cases of aseptic meningitis was smaller overseas than that in Japan. In Canada, by September 1987, aseptic meningitis had developed in 3 children given the dose of a MMR vaccine using the Urabe Am-9 strain after the vaccination. Additional 8 cases were reported by November 1988. In Canada, the vaccine producing companies immediately discontinued manufacture and marketing of the vaccine.

In Japan also, over a period of 1983 through 1989, i.e. even prior to and just after the approval granted for manufacture of and the launch onto the market of the MMR vaccine concerned, there had been 13 case reports for which the occurrences of meningitis after administration of mumps vaccines or the MMR vaccine were suspected to have been related to the vaccination. The company that produced the bulk liquid of mumps vaccine for the problematic product had data regarding health damage, and the data indicated the following: as of December 1989, meningitis had developed in at least 19 vaccinated children; and the PCR method already available at that time revealed that these cases were not caused by the wild strain of mumps but related to the strain derived from the mumps vaccine. This information was neither published nor shared among healthcare professionals.

In 1989, the Maebashi Medical Association in Maebashi City collected data regarding adverse drug reactions since the start of immunization with the MMR vaccine concerned, on the basis of the following consideration: since some children who experience natural infection of mumps may suffer from meningitis, it is expected that administration of live vaccine for mumps could cause the same adverse effect as that in the natural course of infection. The data collection revealed occurrences of meningitis in one per 217 children given the MMR vaccine. These results were reported to the Ministry of Health and Welfare, but as in the above-stated case, this information was neither published nor shared among healthcare professionals. As a result of the combination of these unfortunate circumstances, neither physicians conducting vaccinations, the national government nor parents of children in the designated age range for the vaccination imagined the occurrence of meningitis caused by the MMR vaccine. At last, secondary infection with the MMR vaccine was reported in 1993. Administration of the MMR vaccine was discontinued in 1993.

The Relief System for Injury to Health with Vaccination was applied to 1,065 children who suffered from the MMR vaccine-induced adverse effects. Apart from the relief benefits under this System, the victims filed a lawsuit against the national government and the vaccine manufacturer. The District Court ordered the defendants to pay compensatory damages to the plaintiffs by adjudicating as follows: "It was evident that the manufacturer changed the manufacturing process for the vaccine concerned without notice, and the national government had an obligation to instruct the manufacturer to observe the Pharmaceutical Affairs Law".

MMRワクチン事件に学ぶ

　MMRワクチンは風疹，麻疹，おたふくかぜの3種類の混合ワクチンですが，ワクチンメーカー3社が独自に開発した「独自株ワクチン」が承認されていたにもかかわらず，厚生省が指導してメーカーそれぞれから1種類の原液を交換して混合する「統一株ワクチン」を製造させました。統一株ワクチンでは，他社が製造したワクチン原液の品質管理が困難になるとともに，他社が製造段階で薬事法違反をしてもわかりませんでした。統一株ワクチンを指導した行政の意図は不明ですが，製造工程を複雑にしたことがワクチンに品質問題を生じさせたことと無関係ではない可能性があります。

　MMRワクチンによる無菌性髄膜炎事件とそれに続くMMRワクチン接種の中止は，国民の予防接種に対する信頼を損ない，麻疹に対する予防接種率も低下させ，先進国では例外的に麻疹患者の発生が増加しました。結果として，多くの乳幼児が麻疹そのもので死亡しました。予防接種は公衆衛生の有力な手段であるだけに，その失敗は重大な影響を及ぼします。

　日本ではMMRワクチン事件以外にも予防接種による薬害と言える健康被害があり，定期接種による被害については予防接種健康被害救済制度により，任意接種による健康被害については医薬品副作用被害救済制度により救済されるようになっています。

Lessons learned from the MMR vaccine incident

The MMR vaccine is a "3-in-1" vaccine that protects against rubella, measles, and mumps. The 3 vaccine manufacturers had independently developed "unique strain" for the respective diseases and obtained the approval for their respective vaccines using the unique strains. Despite this fact, under the directions by the Ministry of Health and Welfare, each of the 3 vaccine manufacturers provided a single bulk liquid for the vaccine they produced to the other 2 companies, and then each mixed the 3 bulk liquids to produce the MMR vaccine using the "unified strain". It was difficult for the manufacturers to control the quality of the bulk vaccine liquids produced and provided by the other companies. In addition, even if some of the 3 companies violated the Pharmaceutical Affairs Law, the remaining partner(s) had no way to identify such violation. Although the reason why the Ministry of Health and Welfare guided the companies to produce the MMR vaccine using the unified strain was unknown, this guidance made the vaccine manufacturing processes more complicated, which might have been somewhat related to the development of quality-related problems with the vaccine.

The occurrence of MMR vaccine-induced aseptic meningitis and the subsequent discontinuation of administration of the MMR vaccine damaged public confidence in preventive vaccination, and decreased the rate of preventive vaccination against measles, exceptionally increasing the number of patients with measles to high levels among the developed countries. Consequently, many infants and children have died of measles itself. Since preventive vaccination is an effective public health tool, a failure in the immunization program has a significant impact.

In Japan, preventive vaccination caused health damage events, which may be regarded as drug-induced sufferings, in addition to the MMR vaccine incident. There are two types of vaccinations in Japan, i.e. periodic vaccinations specified in the Preventive Vaccination Law and voluntary vaccinations, and the systems for relief services are in operation as follows: relief benefits for health damage caused by periodic vaccinations are provided under the Relief System for Injury to Health with Vaccination, and relief benefits for health damage caused by voluntary vaccinations are provided under the Relief System for Adverse Drug Reactions.

12　ソリブジン事件

事件の概要

　ソリブジンは日本で開発された優れた抗ウイルス剤で，帯状疱疹を効能として1993年に承認されました。この事件では，ソリブジンとフルオロウラシル系抗がん剤(5-FU)の併用により，重篤な骨髄抑制が発症し，そのため販売開始後1か月で15名の死亡者が出ました。

　ソリブジンはチミジンの類似化合物です。したがって薬理的には，フルオロウラシル系抗がん剤の代謝を核酸系の薬物が阻害して，抗がん剤の血中濃度を高めるということが容易に予測されます。実際にフルオロウラシル系抗がん剤の有効性を持続させるために，代謝を核酸系薬剤で阻害するという動物実験に関する論文がベルギーで出されていました。しかし製薬企業はこの論文を入手していながら，薬物相互作用の検討を十分に行っていませんでした。さらに厚生省はこの論文が承認申請資料として提出されていたにもかかわらず，その危険性を審査段階で見抜けませんでした。

　ソリブジンは開発段階(第Ⅱ相臨床試験)で，フルオロウラシル系抗がん剤との併用によると考えられる死亡例が3例発生していました。また，ラットを用いた併用試験では全例が死亡していました。それにもかかわらず発売時の添付文書には，「フルオロウラシル系抗がん剤との併用を避けること」という相互作用に関する一般的注意にとどまり，警告とはなっていませんでした。

　健康被害の発生は急なものでしたが行政の対応は早く，1993年9月3日に発売，10月8日には企業からの副作用報告を受けて直ちに緊急安全性情報配布を指示，10月12日には報道機関へ発表，11月1日には企業の自主回収となりました。この事件は裁判に発展しませんでしたが，この速やかな対応もその一因だったと考えられます。

　ソリブジンは薬害と言われながらも厚生省は，抗ウイルス剤としての有用性から適正使用の徹底を条件として承認の取り消しをせず，企業の自主回収によって被害は終息しました。そのため，併用禁止のための安全対策を強化すれば，再発売が可能でした。しかし，この事件に製薬企業のインサイダー取引が絡んだこともあり，企業が自主的に承認を取り下げ，ソリブジンは市場から消えることとなりました。

12 Sorivudine Incident

Summary of the incident

Sorivudine was an excellent antiviral agent developed in Japan. It was approved for the indication of herpes zoster in 1993. In the sorivudine incident, concomitant administration of sorivudine and a fluorouracil anticancer agent (5-FU) resulted in 15 deaths due to serious myelosuppression within one month after the launch of sorivudine onto the Japanese market.

Sorivudine was a synthetic analogue of thymidine. From the pharmacological point of view, it is predictable that the metabolism of fluorouracil anticancer agents is inhibited by synthetic analogues of nucleic acids, increasing blood concentrations of the anticancer agents. A paper on animal studies in which metabolism of the fluorouracil anticancer agents was inhibited by nucleic acid analogues with the aim of maintaining the efficacy of the anticancer agents had already been published in Belgium. The company that developed sorivudine had obtained this paper but did not adequately investigate drug-drug interactions. Despite the fact that this paper was included in the data submitted with the application for approval for sorivudine, the Ministry of Health and Welfare failed to identify the risk of this metabolism inhibition at the review stage.

During the clinical development of sorivudine (i.e. in phase II clinical trials), 3 patients died for which combined administration of sorivudine with fluorouracil anticancer agents might have been a potential cause. In animal studies using rats given concomitant administration of the two drugs, all animals died. Despite these facts, the package insert of sorivudine upon its launch only gave the statement to "Avoid concomitant administration with fluorouracil anticancer agents", which was within the range of general precaution and was never specifically outlined as a warning.

Once aware of the sudden occurrences of drug-induced health damage, the regulatory authorities promptly took responsive actions. On September 3, 1993, sorivudine was launched onto the Japanese market. Immediately after receipt of reports on the adverse drug reactions from the company, the Ministry of Health and Welfare instructed distribution of an Urgent Safety Information on October 8, and reported the events to the news media on October 12. The company conducted voluntary recall of the drug on November 1. The sorivudine incident did not lead to lawsuits partly because of these prompt actions.

ソリブジン事件に学ぶ

　ソリブジンは優れた抗ウイルス薬でしたが，発売後の対応を誤ったために市場から消えることになりました。治験段階で抗がん剤との相互作用の可能性が文献的に示唆されていたにもかかわらず，開発段階や審査段階において十分な検討がなされなかったこと，ひいては添付文書における併用に対する注意書きが，「併用を避けること」と最小限な記述であったことが事件の要因でした。その理由の一つは，開発企業がもともと医薬品卸企業であり，新薬の開発の経験が少なかったことにもよると思われます。

　ソリブジンの販売についてのみ提携をしていた製薬企業は，有効性や安全性に対する検討していませんでした。ライセンスホルダーと提携する販売企業の責任も再考する必要があります。

　ソリブジンの被害者の中には帯状疱疹のために皮膚科を受診し，服用していた抗がん剤の実物を見せて，併用の危険性について医師に確認したにも関わらず，問題ないとされて服用し，死亡した事例があります。医師が添付文書を読んでいないということを示唆するケースでした。また，ソリブジンの被害者への投薬では，薬局での併用薬チェックをすり抜けていたことも明らかになっています。医薬分業の進展とともに，薬剤師の役割と責任もより厳しく問われることになりました。

　一方，行政の対応は早かったため，早期に事件は終息しました。問題を認識した時点での断固とした行政の対応が，いかに重要であるかを示しました。しかし事件の半年後になっても，大半の医療機関が被害者・遺族に併用による被害の事実を知らせていないことが明らかになりました。行政の強い意向により，被害の事実が被害者，遺族に伝えられた結果，裁判になることなく企業との和解が成立しました。

　併用で問題となった5-FUは，これまで長く使われている抗がん剤でした。しかしこの

The sorivudine incident was considered a drug-induced suffering. Due to the antiviral usefulness of sorivudine, however, the Ministry of Health and Welfare did not cancel the approval for the drug, provided that thorough dissemination of the proper use of the drug to all those concerned was ensured. The company voluntarily recalled the products, making this incident come to an end. It may be possible to restart marketing of the drug after reinforcing safety securing measures to prohibit the combined use of the two drugs. However, since engagement of pharmaceutical companies in insider trading was disclosed, the company withdrew the approval on its own will, making sorivudine no more commercially available.

Lessons learned from the sorivudine incident

Sorivudine was an excellent antiviral agent. The drug was withdrawn from the market because the actions taken after its launch were not adequate. Despite the fact that the literature pointed out the risk of possible drug-drug interactions between sorivudine and the anticancer agents even at the stage of clinical trials of sorivudine, this risk was not adequately investigated during the development period and at the approval review stage. In addition, the precautionary statement regarding co-administration of sorivudine and the anticancer agents in the package insert of the drug was limited to a minimum, i.e. "avoid concomitant administration". These inadequate actions may be related to the background features of the development company that had originally been a wholesaler of drugs and had not accumulated significant experience in the development of new drugs.

There was a pharmaceutical company that only marketed sorivudine under contract. This company did not investigate the efficacy and safety of the drug, which indicates that the responsibilities of marketing companies having a business tie-up with marketing authorization holders need to be reconsidered.

When visiting the dermatology clinic for the treatment of herpes zoster, a sorivudine victim had discussed with the physician the risk of concomitant use of sorivudine and anticancer agents, and had even showed the specific anticancer drugs the victim was taking to the physician, but was told that there were no problems with the co-administration. Unfortunately the victim took the two drugs together and died. This episode indicates that physicians did not read the package insert. Investigation of how the victims concomitantly took sorivudine and anticancer agents revealed that at hospital pharmacies or dispensing pharmacies, the risk of the co-administration of the two drugs was not detected by a check for combination therapy. Along with the advancement of the system that separates prescribing from dispensing drugs, the roles and responsibilities of pharmacists are

事件により，相互作用という問題は，新しいメカニズムの新薬が出るたびに，これまで長く使用されてきた医薬品についても，新たなリスク発生の可能性があるということを示しました。

　ソリブジン事件により治験の充実・強化の必要性が認識され，1996年に薬事法が大幅に改正されました。主な改正点は次のようなものです。
・GCP，GPMSP（Good Post Marketing Surveillance Practice）の法制化，副作用報告等の収集・評価，報告が義務化されました。
・新薬承認審査体制の強化として，新たに国立医薬品食品衛生研究所内に医薬品医療機器審査センター（審査センター）を設立するとともに，医薬品副作用被害救済・研究振興調査機構（略称：医薬品機構）も強化されました。審査センターは医薬品の承認に係る審査の実務部隊としての役割を担うこととなりました。
・医薬品機構では，申請書類等の信頼性調査と治験相談が開始されました。この相談はユーザーフィーに基づくもので，正式な相談とされるものです。
・新GCPに基づいて治験の規制を強化しました。

　さらに，2001年には
・新薬に対する市販直後調査制度が導入されました。これは新薬の発売直後が最もリスクの高い時期であることから，発売後6か月間はすべての納入医療機関に対して，MRが定期的に訪問し，重篤な副作用の発生を把握することにより，市販直後の安全対策強化につなげていく制度です。

severely called into question.

The sorivudine incident soon came to an end because the Ministry of Health and Welfare promptly took responsive actions, indicating the extreme importance for the regulatory authorities to take determined steps so as to handle a problem soon after they recognize it. Even 6 months after the end of the incident, however, it was revealed that most of the medical institutions did not inform the victims and the bereaved of the fact that the adverse drug reaction was caused by the concomitant administration of two drugs. Due to the strong directions by the Ministry of Health and Welfare, this fact was eventually communicated to the victims and the bereaved. As a result of this communication, no lawsuits were filed but settlements out of the courts were agreed upon by the victims and the companies concerned.

The anticancer agent 5-FU, a counterpart of the combination therapy causing this incident, has long been used. This has given the lesson that whenever a new drug with a new mechanism of action becomes available, new risks of drug-drug interactions may be raised even for drugs which have long been used.

The sorivudine incident highlighted the necessity of improving the quality of and reinforcing the framework for clinical trials. In 1996, the Pharmaceutical Affairs Law underwent a major amendment. The main points of this amendment are indicated below.
- Legalization of GCP and GPMSP (Good Post Marketing Surveillance Practice). Making it mandatory to collect, evaluate, and report adverse drug reactions, etc.
- For the purpose of reinforcing the review system for approval of new drugs, the Pharmaceutical and Medical Devices Evaluation Center (PMDEC) was newly established in the National Institute of Health Sciences, and in addition, the Organization for Pharmaceutical Safety and Research (OPSR) was enhanced. The PMDEC has fulfilled practical duties with regards to reviews for approval of drugs.
- The OPSR started to conduct inspections and reliability assessment for the submitted data for applications for approval as well as other relevant documentation and to provide clinical trial consultation services. This consultation is based on users' fees and regarded as an official consultation.
- Intensifying the regulations on clinical trials on the basis of the New GCP

Furthermore, in 2001,
- The early post-marketing phase vigilance (EPPV) system for new drugs was introduced, with the aim of reinforcing risk minimization measures in the early phase after the launch of a new drug, since the risk(s) associated with the use of the new drug is greatest over this early post-marketing

period; for the first 6 months after the start of marketing, medical representatives (MRs) of pharmaceutical companies make periodic visits to all medical institutions to which the new drug is delivered, so as to identify the occurrence of a serious adverse drug reaction, if any, so as to help reinforcing the safety measures in this particular period.

13 ヒト乾燥硬膜による プリオン感染(CJD)事件

事件の概要

　日本における異常プリオンによる医原的感染が明らかになったのは，狂牛病の感染問題を契機にヤコブ病について1996年に緊急調査が全国で行われた時です。当時の日本では，ヤコブ病患者826例のうち43例がドイツからの輸入ヒト乾燥硬膜を移植されていました。その結果，1997年3月，厚生省はヒト乾燥硬膜の使用を禁止にしました。日本ではこの医療機器を1973年に輸入を開始して以来，24年間も使用してきたのです。しかしこの間，1987年に米国では1例の発症事例を以て当該製品が使用禁止となり，全世界に警告が出されました。しかし，日本では使用が継続されました。

　2011年12月現在で133名の患者数が確認されていますが，日本では回収が遅れた上に不徹底だったこともあり，今後も患者数は増える可能性があります。

　1996年に被害者が，国と製造業者及び輸入販売業者を相手取って初めての提訴を行いました。2001年に裁判所の和解勧告により和解が成立しました。当初，国は米国から情報を得た1987年以前には危険性を知りえなかったので責任を回避する主張を行いましたが，最終的には，被害者全員を救済することに合意しました。ヒト硬膜は生体移植を行うものでありながら，医療機器として安易な輸入許可を行ったとされます。

ヒト乾燥硬膜によるプリオン感染事件に学ぶ

　ヒト乾燥硬膜という生物由来製品が，医薬品ではなく医療機器に分類されていました。医薬品については薬害を教訓とした法規制や体制が構築されてきていましたが，医療機

13 Human Dried Dura Mater Induced Prion Infection (CJD) Incident

Summary of the incident

In Japan, it was not until 1996 that iatrogenic transmission of Creutzfeldt-Jakob Disease (CJD) due to prions was identified by a nationwide emergency survey on CJD conducted due to the issue of mad cow disease (bovine spongiform encephalopathy). At the time, there were 826 patients given a diagnosis of CJD in Japan, and of the 826, 43 had received human dried dura mater grafts imported from Germany. In March 1997, the Ministry of Health and Welfare banned the use of human dried dura mater grafts. This means that in Japan, these medical devices had been used for as long as 24 years since the start of import in 1973. In the US, however, the use of the product concerned was banned in 1987 on the basis of one case of the product-induced disease, and the warning was distributed all over the world. Despite this warning, use of the responsible product was continued in Japan.

As of December 2011, 133 patients with the disease were identified. In Japan, however, since the recall of the product concerned was delayed and was not conducted thoroughly, the number of patients may continue to increase from now on.

In 1996, a victim first filed a lawsuit against the national government, the drug manufacturing company, and the company that imported and marketed the drug. In 2001, the courts recommended a settlement and the defendants accepted the court-brokered settlement. The national government originally claimed that the state was not liable for this issue because they had not been able to be aware of the risk prior to 1987 when they obtained the information from the US. However, the state eventually agreed on provision of relief benefits to all victims. Despite the fact that transplantation of human dura mater graft was exactly the same as implementation of living donor organ transplantation, the national government gave its approval for import of the dura mater product concerned as a medical device without reviewing it comprehensively.

Lessons learned from the human dried dura mater induced prion infection (CJD) incident

The human dried dura mater, a biological product, was included not in the category of drugs but in that of medical devices. For drugs, the laws and regulations as well as regulatory systems had been

に関しては未整備でした．また，医療機器の輸入販売企業の意識も医薬品業界に比べて相当に立ち遅れていました．ヒト乾燥硬膜の輸入販売企業はプリオン感染の可能性を知りながら，厚生省に報告して製造方法の一部変更を行わず，不活化処理も不十分でした．また，国立予防衛生研究所の職員がCDCによる警告の事実を知って専門誌に投稿したにも関わらず，本省の担当部局に連絡していなかったことが明らかになっています．組織間，組織内における情報の共有の重要さは強調しすぎることはありません．

この事件は20年近くも前に輸入承認されたヒト材料が原因となったもので，行政における審査や安全対策の担当官は，このような製品が大量に使用されていることをほとんど認識していなかったとされます．また，世界で生産されるヒト硬膜製品の半分が日本に輸入されていました．医原性CJDのほとんどが，日本国内だけで報告されていることと符合します．日本での需要が突出していることは，血液製剤でも同様でした．ヒト由来の製品は極めて貴重な資源であるとともに，臓器移植に伴う危険性もあるという認識が医療現場に不足しているのではないかと考えられます．

本製品はドイツからの輸入でしたが，外国製造業者，輸入販売業者ともに製造管理と安全性確保において杜撰であったことが判明しました．生物由来製品の安全管理は2002年の薬事法改正で強化され，外国製造業者に対するGMP査察は2005年から施行されました．プリオン感染が特異であることから，手術現場における衛生，汚染管理について厚生省から管理のガイドラインが出されました．

established on the basis of the lessons learned from previous drug-induced sufferings. For medical devices, however, these establishments had not been adequately formulated. In addition, the companies importing and marketing medical devices were insufficiently aware of what they had to do as marketers, as compared with those handling drugs. The company that imported and marketed the human dried dura mater did know the potential risk of prion infection, but neither reported it to the Ministry of Health and Welfare nor made an application for approval for change in the approved manufacturing method to the regulatory authorities. Furthermore, their inactivation treatment of the product was inadequate. It was revealed that the staff at the National Institute of Health in Japan became aware of the warning issued by the US Centers for Disease Control and Prevention (CDC) and contributed this fact to a specialist periodical, but failed to inform the responsible division of the Ministry of Health and Welfare. This again highlights how important it is to share information between relevant functions and within individual functions.

CJD suffering was caused by human-derived materials imported as long as 20 years ago, at which time the government officials responsible for review and safety measures rarely recognized that human dura mater grafts were used in large quantities in Japan. At that time, almost half the human dura mater products manufactured over the world were imported to Japan. This is in agreement with the fact that almost all cases of iatrogenic transmission of CJD were reported in Japan only. The prominent consumption in Japan was noted also for blood products. These facts may serve to indicate that the healthcare professionals in medical settings are insufficiently aware that products made from raw materials of human origin are extremely valuable resources and also involve risks associated with organ transplantation.

The product that caused the CJD incident in Japan was imported from Germany. Investigation revealed that both the German manufacturer and the Japanese importing and marketing company exercised insufficient care in production control and securing safety. The amendment of the Pharmaceutical Affairs Law in 2002 reinforced the safety control for biological products. The GMP inspection on foreign manufacturers was started in 2005. Since prion infection is specific, the Ministry of Health and Welfare formulated guidelines on hygiene and contamination control in operating rooms.

14 ウシ心嚢膜抗酸菌様感染事件

事件の概要

　ウシ心嚢膜は，開胸手術における心筋保護などを目的として使われました。ヒト乾燥硬膜と同様に事件当時は，医療機器として扱われていた米国からの輸入製品でした。問題となった製品は，1987年に米国からの輸入が承認されていたものです。

　1999年10月，複数の医療機関から代用心膜として使われた患者で遅発性無菌性皮下膿症（縦隔炎）の発症が厚生省へ報告されました。同年12月，厚生省は原因の特定はできないものの，本製品を代用心膜として使用しないよう医療機関に注意喚起を行いました。翌2000年1月には米国FDAに，ウシ心嚢膜に関して照会を行いました。ウシ心嚢膜を泌尿器関係の手術に使用した後，遅発性の化膿状態になったケースが複数あることが回答されましたが同時に，FDAは特段の措置を取らないことも報告されました。

　同年2月には輸入業者より，保存サンプルから抗酸菌が検出されたとの報告があり，3月には患者の生体試料より抗酸菌が検出されました。これにより厚生省は輸入業者に対して，医療機関への追加情報の提供，患者のフォローアップの徹底及び因果関係究明を指示しました。

　さらに同年9月，厚生省はそれまで把握，検討した以下の情報を医療機関に提供しました。
・使用枚数は3,156枚，使用施設137施設，健康被害は13施設で，合計62例の遅発性皮下膿症が発症。発症までの期間は1〜51週間。
・国内3施設で原因菌の同定を試みたが，培養が困難であり，同定には至らず。

　その後2001年3月までに，原因究明が進みました。一部の製品と患者から摘出した製品より同一のDNAパターンのサルモネラ菌が検出され，さらに未使用の製品のすべてから1〜2種類の菌が検出されました。菌は製品の表面ではなく内部から検出されており，深部に潜在していた菌が使用後に表面に移行して感染，発症したことが推定されました。これにより，同製品は2001年に販売中止となりました。

14 Incident of Bovine Pericardium Induced Infection with Probably Acid-Fast Bacilli

Summary of the incident

Bovine pericardial patches were used for myocardial protection during open heart surgery. Like the human dried dura mater graft, bovine pericardium was included in the category of medical devices when the suffering due to these patches occurred. The product causing this incident was imported from the US and obtained a Japanese official approval for import in 1987.

In October 1999, several medical institutions reported to the Ministry of Health and Welfare (MHW) that delayed aseptic subcutaneous abscess (mediastinitis) developed in patients for whom bovine pericardial patches had been used as a substitute pericardium. In December 1999, although the cause of the adverse event was not identified, the MHW called the attention of staff at medical institutions so as to ensure that the product concerned was not used as a substitute pericardium. In January 2000, the MHW made an inquiry to the US FDA, which gave its answer that in multiple cases, delayed purulence developed after bovine pericardial patches had been used in urological operations. The FDA also answered that they did not take any special measures to handle this matter.

In February 2000, the Japanese importer reported to the MHW that acid-fast bacilli were detected in the samples they stored. In March 2000, the bacteria were detected in patients' biospecimens. The MHW then directed the importer to provide additional information to the medical institutions, to conduct thorough follow-up of patients, and to try to identify a causal relationship between the product concerned and the adverse event.

In September 2000, the MHW provided the information listed below that they had obtained and evaluated by that time, to the medical institutions.
- A total of 3,156 patches were used in 137 medical institutions. The health hazard occurred in 13 medical institutions. A total of 62 patients with delayed subcutaneous abscess were identified. The length of time until the onset of the event ranged from one to 51 weeks.
- In 3 medical institutions in Japan, identification of causative organisms was attempted. However, since culturing was difficult, identification was unsuccessful.

ウシ心嚢膜抗酸菌様感染事件に学ぶ

　ヒト硬膜によるCJD事件と同様に，本事件も医療機器として分類，取り扱われていた製品によるものです。被害の規模も限定的で薬害事件としての社会的な認知度はほとんどありませんが，薬事規制上は生物由来製品による健康被害リスクを考えさせるきっかけとなりました。健康被害の報告から販売中止まで比較的短期間で推移しましたが，CJD事件と同様に輸入品であること，医療機器に分類されていたことから原因究明には試行錯誤が必要でした。

　この事件の教訓は2002年の薬事法改正に生かされ，生物由来製品の製造管理の強化，外国製造所に対するGMP査察強化として反映されました。バイオテクノロジーの発展による医療技術の進歩に対して，そのリスクの増大も十分に考慮する必要があります。

Subsequently, the exploration of the cause was ongoing until March 2001. Salmonella isolated from some of the products and from the products that were extracted from the patients had identical DNA patterns. In addition, from all unused products that were examined, one or two species of bacteria were detected. The bacteria were detected not from the product surface but from the inside of the products, suggesting that the bacteria had colonized the deep part of the product, moved up to the surface after the product was used, and caused the infection and the health hazard. In 2001, marketing of this responsible product was discontinued.

Lessons learned from the incident of bovine pericardium induced infection with probably acid-fast bacilli

As in the case of human dried dura mater graft-induced CJD, the bovine pericardium that was handled as a medical device was responsible for the suffering, although the scale of which was limited. The bovine pericardium induced infection is little recognized by society as a drug-induced suffering, but provoked an important opportunity from the viewpoint of pharmaceutical regulatory system, i.e. consideration of potential health hazard risks associated with biological products. Marketing of the responsible patch product was discontinued in a relatively short period of time since the report of the health hazard. As in the case of the CJD incident, trial and error was necessary to identify the cause since the responsible product was imported from overseas and was included in the category of medical devices.

The lessons from this incident were effectively utilized in the amendment of the Pharmaceutical Affairs Law in 2002, i.e. reinforcement of manufacturing management of biological products, and enhancement of GMP inspection to foreign manufacturing establishment. As biotechnology advances, it is required to give full consideration to increasing risks associated with the advancement in medical care.

15 ゲフィチニブ事件

事件の概要

　ゲフィチニブ(販売名：イレッサ)は世界で初めて，2002年7月に日本で承認された，治療法の少ない非小細胞肺がんを効能とした，分子標的薬です。従来の細胞毒性をもつ抗がん剤とメカニズムが異なるため，副作用が少なく，効果の高い新薬として承認が待たれていました。このためゲフィチニブは優先審査で承認され，薬価基準収載の前から特定療養費扱いで使用が認められるという，特例扱いでした。患者，医師，専門家，行政もその期待は大きく，マスコミで大きく繰り返し取り上げられました。

　ゲフィチニブの健康被害は，7月に承認された直後の発売時から重篤な肺障害，とりわけ間質性肺炎となって現れました。間質性肺炎については開発の段階で認められており，発売時の添付文書にも記載されていました。しかし使用が拡大するにつれ，重篤な副作用の報告も急激に増加することとなり，2002年の10月には緊急安全性情報が出され，添付文書には警告欄が設けられました。

緊急安全性情報(2002年10月)

1. 急性肺障害，間質性肺炎が現れることがあるので，胸部X線検査などを行うなど，観察を十分に行い，異常が認められた場合には投与を中止し，適切な処置を行う
2. 急性肺障害，間質性肺炎などの重篤な副作用が起こることがあり，致命的な経過をたどることがあるので，臨床症状(呼吸状態，咳および発熱等の有無)を十分観察し，定期的に胸部X線検査を行う
3. 必要に応じて胸部CT検査，動脈血酸素分圧(PaO_2)，肺胞気動脈血酸素分圧格差($A-aDO_2$)，肺拡張能力(DLco)などの検査を行い，急性肺障害，間質性肺炎などが疑われた場合には，直ちに本剤による治療を中止し，ステロイド治療などの適切な処置をおこなう
4. 本剤の副作用について患者に十分説明するとともに，臨床症状(息切れ，呼吸困難，咳および発熱等の有無)を十分に観察し，これらが発現した場合には速やかに医療機関を受診するように患者を指導

添付文書改訂
警告欄に上記1.を，使用上の注意の「重要な基本的注意」に2. 3. 4を記載し，医療関係者に対し注意喚起

15 Gefitinib Incident

Summary of the incident

Gefitinib (trade name: Iressa), a molecular targeted drug, was approved in Japan first in the world in July 2002 for the indication of non-small cell lung cancer, for which only a small number of therapies are available. Since its mechanism of action is different from those of the existing cytotoxic anticancer agents, this new drug was expected to be highly effective and associated with fewer adverse reactions. Its approval was eagerly awaited. For this reason gefitinib was handled as a special: it was subject to the Priority Review for approval, and even before its inclusion in the National Health Insurance (NHI) drug price listing, its use was permitted under the Special Healthcare Expenditure System. Patients, medical doctors, specialists, and the administrative organization had great expectation on gefitinib. The new drug repeatedly received prominent coverage in the mass media.

At the time of the launch of gefitinib onto the market immediately after its approval in July 2002, serious lung disorder, especially interstitial pneumonia, occurred as a drug-induced health damage. The development of interstitial pneumonia had been noted in the clinical development of the drug and was stated in the package insert distributed at the time of its launch. However, as the use of the drug was more widespread, the number of reports on serious adverse drug reactions rapidly increased. In October 2002, an Urgent Safety Information was issued and a column of warning(s) was established in the package insert.

Urgent Safety Information (October 2002)

1. Since acute lung disorder and interstitial pneumonia may occur, observe patients carefully, e.g. by performing chest X-ray examination. If any abnormality is identified, discontinue the administration and take appropriate actions to treat such event.
2. Since serious adverse drug reactions including, among others, acute lung disorder and interstitial pneumonia, may occur and such reaction may be fatal, observe patients for clinical symptoms (the status of respiration, the presence or absence of cough, fever, etc.) with vigilance and perform chest X-ray examination periodically.
3. As appropriate, perform chest CT examination and determine partial pressure of oxygen in arterial blood (PaO_2), alveolar-arterial difference in oxygen tension (A-aDO_2), diffusion capacity of lungs for carbon monoxide (DLco), and other relevant tests. If acute lung disorder or interstitial pneumonia is suspected, immediately discontinue the treatment with gefitinib and administer appropriate therapy such as steroids to treat such event.

しかし，その後もゲフィチニブの使用の増加に伴い，間質性肺炎発症の報告は止まりませんでした。そのため厚生労働省は，12月に専門家会議を開催した結果，警告の内容を強化し，少なくとも投与開始後4週間は入院もしくはそれに準じる管理の下に置くことを義務づけました。ゲフィチニブは錠剤であり，1日1回投与で家庭での投薬が可能であったため，患者が変調を感じても受診しなければ医師は対処ができないこと，また間質性肺炎という健康被害が原疾患の増悪と区別しがたいため，患者自身の対応が遅れることへの対処でした。

　また，医療機関も選別されることとなりました。しかし当時，日本にはがん化学療法の専門家は限られており，学会としてのガイドラインも作成されていませんでした。

警告欄の追加記載

1. 副作用についての患者への説明と同意を得ること
2. 急性肺障害や間質性肺炎が本剤の投与の初期に発生し，致命的な転帰をたどる例が多いため，少なくとも投与開始後4週間は入院またはそれに準ずる管理の下で，間質性肺炎などの重篤な副作用発現に関する観察を十分におこなうこと
3. 肺がん化学療法に十分な経験を持つ医師が使用するとともに，投与に際しては緊急時に十分措置できる医療機関で行うこと

　以上の安全対策を強化して適正使用の徹底を図った結果，その後の有害事象の報告は大幅に低下しました。ゲフィチニブは，ソリブジン事件の教訓から制定された市販直後調査の対象となる第一号の新薬でした。厚生労働省は副作用が拡大していく過程で，薬事法に

> 4. Give thorough explanation of the adverse reaction of gefitinib to patients. In addition, observe patients for clinical symptoms (the presence or absence of breath shortness, dyspnea, cough, fever, etc.). Instruct patients to make a prompt visit to medical institutions whenever any of such symptoms occurs.
>
> **Revision of the package insert**
> The statement in Item 1 above was entered in the column of warning(s), and Items 2, 3, and 4, in the subsection of "Important Precaution(s)" of the section "PRECAUTIONS", so as to raise awareness of healthcare professionals about these matters.

Nevertheless, the spread of gefitinib treatment still continued thereafter and reports on the development of interstitial pneumonia persisted. In December 2002, the Ministry of Health, Labour and Welfare held a meeting of an experts committee, which decided to reinforce the warnings and made it mandatory to hospitalize patients or place them under the similar control to hospitalization for at least 4 weeks after the start of treatment with gefitinib. These actions were aimed at handling the following situations: since gefitinib was in tablet form and taken once daily by patients at home, abnormalities which patients noticed were not treated by physicians unless they visited clinics or hospitals; and since interstitial pneumonia, the adverse reaction of the drug, was difficult to differentiate from worsening of the underlying disease, patients themselves delayed taking adequate actions to cope with the event.

Furthermore, it was decided to start specifically selecting medical institutions performing gefitinib treatment. At that time in Japan, however, there were only a limited number of specialists in chemotherapy of cancer and no guidelines were issued by the relevant academic societies or associations.

> **Additional entries in the column of warning(s)**
>
> 1. Regarding the adverse drug reactions, give thorough explanation to patients and obtain informed consent from them.
> 2. Acute lung disorder or interstitial pneumonia may occur soon after the start of treatment with gefitinib, resulting in fatal outcome in many cases. Hospitalize patients or place them under the similar control to hospitalization for at least 4 weeks after the start of treatment, during which patients shall carefully be observed for possible occurrences of serious adverse drug reactions such as interstitial pneumonia.
> 3. Only those physicians with extensive experience in chemotherapy for lung cancer shall use gefitinib. Furthermore, gefitinib therapy shall be administered at medical institutions where adequate actions will be taken in case of emergency.

As stated above, the drug safety measures were reinforced and attempts were made to fully disseminate the proper use of gefitinib to the healthcare professionals concerned, which substantially reduced the number of reports on adverse events. Gefitinib was the first new drug that

基づく企業への立ち入り検査を行いましたが，企業の規制遵守状況に問題は見られませんでした。

ゲフィチニブの健康被害は裁判に発展しました。裁判の争点は，企業に対しては発売時の添付文書の記載内容の妥当性及び，国の添付文書記載に対する指導責任が問われました。裁判は最高裁まで上訴されましたが，企業及び国に責任がないことが確定しました。

ゲフィチニブ事件に学ぶもの

ゲフィチニブ事件は発売前の状況という点で，その9年前に起きたソリブジン事件と共通するものがあります。ゲフィチニブは分子標的薬という従来の細胞毒性型の抗がん剤とは違うメカニズムから副作用が少なく，また肺がんという治療困難な疾病に対して内服で使用できるという，前評判と期待が先行した薬でした。分子標的薬の抗がん剤として世界で最初に日本で承認した薬として，行政，企業，医療従事者，患者のすべてが有効性に目を奪われていたということは否定できない状況でした。このため，ゲフィチニブ事件はソリブジンと同様に短期間で非常に多くの患者に使用され，急速に被害が拡大したことが挙げられます。ソリブジン事件と同様に，発売前の期待が大きいということは，被害がいったん発生すると急速に拡大する条件が整うということが言えます。

ゲフィチニブはソリブジン事件の教訓から制定された市販直後調査の対象となった第一号の新薬でしたが，急速な健康被害の拡大に安全対策は後手に回りました。発売に備えて，事前の十分な安全対策の構築が必要であることを示した事例でした。緊急安全性情報の発出と間質性肺炎や肺障害等に特化した添付文書の改訂だけでは被害の抑制には十分でなく，2か月後に再度添付文書の改訂を行い，入院により管理すること及び肺がんの化学療法の専門家が使用することを義務付ける必要がありました。

間質性肺炎を含む重篤な事象は発売時の添付文書に記載されていました。その記載が不十分であるかが後日，裁判の焦点となりました。裁判で添付文書に問題ないことが確定しましたが，結果として薬害に発展したことは規制，基準にあるいは法令に適合することと安全対策が機能することとは別物であることを示しました。

ゲフィチニブが医療現場で安易に使われたことも識者によって指摘されています。欧米での使用実績がなく，まったく新しい医薬品で肺がんという重篤な疾病を適用とする薬で

was subject to the early post-marketing phase vigilance (EPVV), a system introduced on the basis of the lessons from the sorivudine incident. As the adverse drug reaction of gefitinib increased, the Ministry of Health, Labour and Welfare conducted on-the-spot inspections at the company concerned and found no problems with the company's compliance with the regulations.

The gefitinib-induced health damage brought about lawsuits. The focal point of the trial was the appropriateness of what was stated in the package insert of gefitinib when it was put on sale and the national government's responsibility to have the drug company provide sufficient information about the relevant matters in the package insert. The lower court's rulings were appealed to the Supreme Court, which absolved the Japanese government and the company of the liability.

Lessons learned from the gefitinib incident

The gefitinib incident had some common pre-launch situations to the sorivudine incident that occurred 9 years earlier. Since gefitinib is a molecular targeted drug and had a different mechanism of action from the cytotoxic anticancer agents existing at the time, the drug was the focus of much interest and expectation even prior to its launch onto the market; gefitinib would be associated with fewer adverse reactions and could be administered as an oral therapy to treat lung cancer, which is usually difficult to treat. In other words, it is not an exaggeration to state that the efficacy of gefitinib that was approved in Japan, the first in the world, as a molecular targeted anticancer agent, fascinated all stakeholders, including the administrative organization, the company, healthcare professionals, and patients. Under these circumstances, as in the sorivudine incident, gefitinib was used by an extremely large number of patients within a short period of time, resulting in a rapid expansion of the damage. The two incidents highlight that great expectation on a drug prior to its launch onto the market set up conditions under which once a drug-induced health damage occurs, it rapidly expands.

Gefitinib was the first new drug subject to the early post-marketing phase vigilance (EPPV) system that was established on the basis of the lessons from the sorivudine incident. However, since the health damage so rapidly expanded, the safety measures were not implemented in time. This incident underlines the need for establishing adequate and sufficient safety measures for a new drug prior to its launch onto the market. The damage related to gefitinib was not adequately controlled by the issuance of the Urgent Safety Information or by the revision of the package insert with special regards to interstitial pneumonia and lung disorder. The package insert was revised again two months later so as to make it mandatory to hospitalize patients on gefitinib treatment with the aim of controlling them adequately and to have specialists in lung cancer chemotherapy use gefitinib.

▶厚生労働省に報告されているイレッサ錠使用との関連が疑われている急性肺障害・間質性肺炎の副作用の発現状況(4月22日現在)

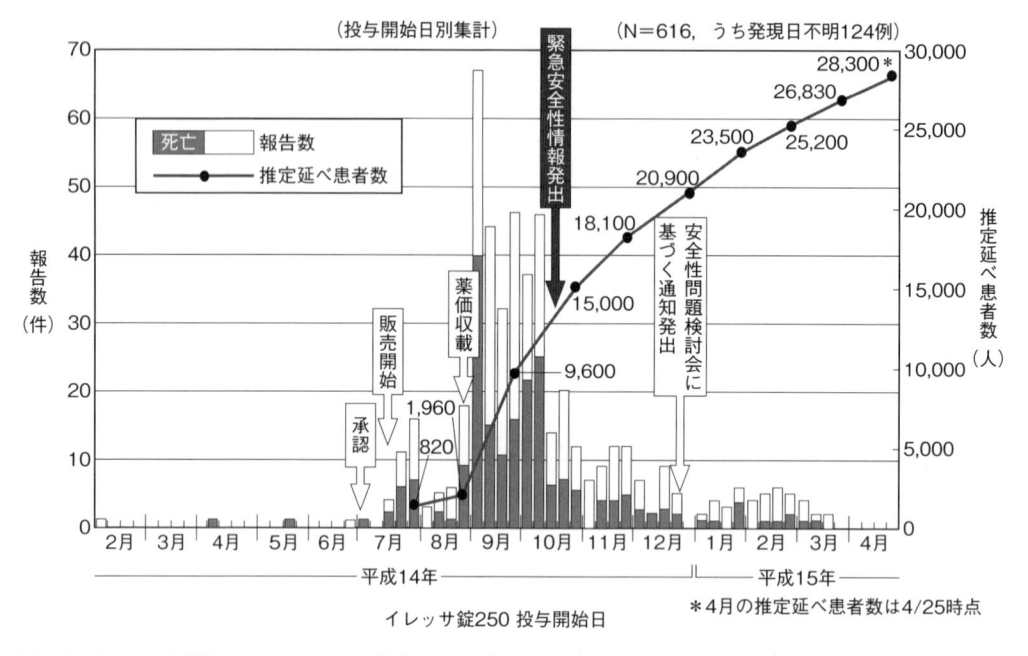

[平成15年5月2日 厚生労働省ゲフィチニブ安全性問題検討会資料から：http://www.mhlw.go.jp/shingi/2003/05/dl/s0502-1d.pdf]

は，そのリスクを見極めつつ医療現場に浸透させていくことが重要です。そのためには医療機関の限定や全例調査などの承認条件を付与する慎重さが必要でした。全例調査は，納入医療機関で使用されるすべての症例について調査票を用いた調査を行うもので，これが実施されていれば，急速な被害拡大は防ぎえたのではないかと考えられます。事実，ゲフィチニブ事件を契機として全例調査が承認条件とされた品目数は，その後，急速に増えました（4章参照のこと）。

　もう一つ，ゲフィチニブの肺障害に対する危険性は審査段階で指摘されていました。しかし，その審査報告書が公表されたのは事件が発生した後のことでした。当時，日本においてはがん治療の専門医制度はなく，抗がん剤治療のガイドラインもありませんでした。審査報告書は企業の立場とは異なる視点で薬のプロファイルを評価しています。医療従事者に対して，企業の立場からだけでない情報提供も担保する必要があると考えられます。審査報告書の内容が適切な時期に公表されていれば，企業の安全対策あるいは医療側の認識にも影響を与えていた可能性があったと考えられます。

▶ Occurrences of lung disorder and interstitial pneumonia, the adverse drug reactions, reported to the Ministry of Health, Labour and Welfare, for which a relation to the use of Iressa tablets was suspected (as of April 22)

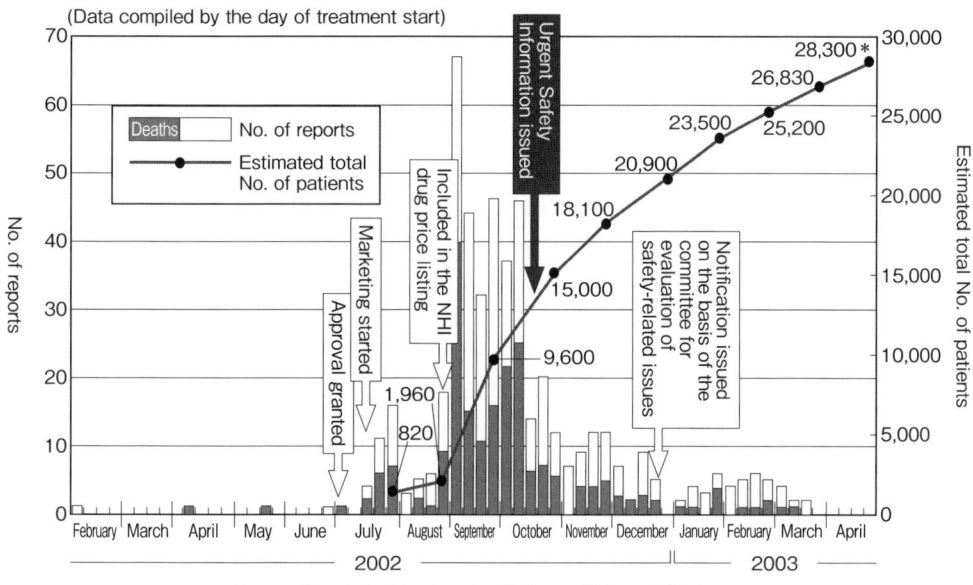

(n=616; For 124 of the 616 patients, the day on which the adverse drug reactions occurred was unknown.)

[Derived from the data distributed at a meeting of the committee for evaluation of gefitinib safety-related issues held on May 2, 2003 : http://www.mhlw.go.jp/shingi/2003/05/dl/s0502-1d.pdf]

The possible onset of serious adverse events including interstitial pneumonia was stated in the package insert at the time of the launch of gefitinib onto the market. The lawsuits were filed later and whether or not the information given in the package insert sufficiently warned against the possibility of these events was the issue of the trial. The court judged that there were no defects with respect to the information stated in the package insert. However, in reality, the occurrence of the gefitinib related serious adverse reactions ultimately developed into an incident of drug-induced suffering. This fact indicates that compliance with regulations, standards, or laws and ordinances is a different issue from having safety measures function adequately.

Knowledgeable people have pointed out that gefitinib was used in actual clinical settings easily or without profound consideration. If a drug has never been used in European and North American countries prior to its use in Japan and is a very novel medication to treat lung cancer, a serious disease, then it is important to ensure that use of the drug is spread stepwise while identifying possible risks to the drug and making sure that adequate safety measures are taken. In the case of

さらに，厚生労働省は審査段階で肺障害発生の可能性を指摘していました．しかし，発売後の被害拡大に対する緊急安全性情報の発出の指示や，追加の安全対策の指示が遅れ，ソリブジン事件の教訓が活かされませんでした．

gefitinib, more caution should have been exercised, e.g. by allowing limited medical institutions to use gefitinib or by requiring all-patient post-marketing surveillance as a condition for approval for gefitinib. All-patient post-marketing surveillance is to investigate all patients treated with a drug at all medical institutions to which the drug is delivered. If this surveillance had been conducted for gefitinib, rapid expansion of the damage could have been avoided. In fact, following the gefitinib incident, the number of drug products to which implementation of all-patient post-marketing surveillance is required as a condition for approval has dramatically increased (see Chapter 4).

Another point to mention is that the risk of development of lung disorder caused by gefitinib had been raised during the review for approval for the drug. The written report on official review for the drug was only made public after the gefitinib incident had occurred. At that time, Japan had no medical specialist system for cancer therapy and no guidelines for anti-cancer therapy. A report on official review evaluates a drug profile from the different viewpoints from those of the company concerned. It may be necessary to provide healthcare professionals with information obtained from different perspective from that of the relevant company. If the information contained in the report on official review for gefitinib had been released to the public at an adequate timing, it may have had an influence on the safety measures taken by the responsible company and the understanding of the issue on the side of healthcare providers.

Furthermore, the Ministry of Health, Labour and Welfare pointed out the possible occurrence of gefitinib related lung disorder at the stage of approval review for the drug. However, they did not instruct in a timely manner issuance of the Urgent Safety Information in response to the post-marketing rapid expansion of health damage and implementation of additional safety measures. The lessons from the sorivudine incidence were not applied.

chapter 3

日本の薬害事件の概括と分析

OVERVIEW AND ANALYSIS OF DRUG-INDUCED SUFFERING IN JAPAN

1. 日本の薬害と薬事制度の変遷と特徴

第2章で，私たちは15件の薬害事件を取り上げました。ここではそれらに加えて，それ以外の薬害事件と主な健康被害を**表1**に示しました。

第2章でそれぞれの事件の概要を説明しましたが，薬害事件の多くは民事裁判という形で決着すると同時に，その教訓はさまざまな形で日本の薬事制度に反映されてきました。

欧米と異なり，日本の民事裁判では原状回復のために，多くは被害者が国と製薬企業を訴えます。つまり，医療関係者の責任が問われる事例はきわめて少数です。このことが，現在までの日本の医薬品等における安全対策の性格を決めてきたと言えます。裁判などに

表1　戦後の日本で発生した薬害事件および主な健康被害事例

1948年	ジフテリア予防接種禍事件*
1956年	ペニシリンショック事件*
1962年	サリドマイド事件*
1965年	アンプル入り風邪薬事件*
1967年	ストレプトマイシン・カナマイシンによる聴力障害
1968年	クロラムフェニコールによる再生不良性貧血
1969年	クロロキンによる網膜症
1970年	スモン事件*
1970年	種痘禍事件
1973年	筋短縮症事件*
1975年	予防接種（DPT三種混合）事件
1975年	未熟児網膜症事件
1982年	ダイアライザーによる眼障害*
1983年	エイズ事件*
1987年	C型肝炎事件*
1988年	陣痛促進剤事件*
1992年	MMRワクチン事件*
1993年	ソリブジン事件*
1994年	イリノテカンによる骨髄抑制・下痢
1997年	CJD事件*
2000年	ウシ心嚢膜による抗酸菌様感染*
2002年	ゲフィチニブ事件*

＊印は2章で取り上げた事件

1. Drug-Induced Suffering in Japan, and Resulting Changes in the Japanese Pharmaceutical Regulatory System and its Characteristics

Chapter 2 summarizes 15 incidents of drug-induced suffering. Table 1 lists other drug-induced sufferings and major health damage events in addition to the 15 incidents.

As Chapter 2 outlines the individual incidents, many of the drug-induced sufferings came to an end in the form of civil lawsuits. At the same time, the lessons from these incidents have been incorporated into improving the pharmaceutical regulatory system in Japan.

Unlike North American and European countries, in Japan victims in many cases file civil lawsuits against the national government and pharmaceutical companies in order to seek personal

Table 1 Post-war drug-induced sufferings and major health damage events in Japan

Year	Event
1948	Diphtheria immunization incident *
1956	Penicillin shock incident *
1962	Thalidomide incident *
1965	Cold-medicines-in-ampoules incident *
1967	Hearing loss caused by antibiotics such as streptomycin and kanamycin
1968	Aplastic anemia caused by chloramphenicol
1969	Retinopathy caused by chloroquine
1970	SMON incident *
1970	Smallpox vaccine incident
1973	Muscle contracture incident *
1975	Vaccination (a "3-in-1" vaccine against DPT (diphtheria, pertussis, and tetanus)) incident
1975	Retinopathy of prematurity incident
1982	Dialyzer induced ophthalmologic disorders incident *
1983	AIDS incident *
1987	Hepatitis C virus (HCV) infection incident *
1988	Labor-inducing drugs incident *
1992	MMR vaccine incident *
1993	Sorivudine incident *
1994	Bone marrow suppression and diarrhea caused by irinotecan
1997	Human dried dura mater induced prion infection (CJD) incident *
2000	Incident of bovine pericardium induced infection with probably acid-fast bacilli *
2002	Gefitinib incident *

Note that the incidents described in Chapter 2 are marked with * .

おける薬害再発防止の議論は，開発から使用までの各段階における薬事規制の強化に結実しました。行政では，開発から市販後への流れに対する薬事監視の強化および審査・安全対策の体制が強化されました。さらに，医薬品等の健康被害救済制度の導入および生物由来製品による感染等救済制度が整備されました。**表2**は，主な薬害事件の教訓がどのように薬事規制に結び付いたかを要約・整理したものです。

日本では，新薬の市販後の安全性確保には，開発から市販後までの一貫したリスク管理（ライフサイクルリスクマネジメント）が必要であるという考え方に基づき，条件付き承認制度（2002年改正で罰則付きに）や，新薬を対象とした市販直後調査を欧米に先駆けて導入しました。これらの考え方は，ICHにおけるE2Eガイドライン作成の原動力になったと同時に，1990年代においては，日本の安全対策に関する薬事制度は欧米に一歩先んじたものでありました。以下に，日本の薬事制度に特徴的な3点について触れておきます。

第1は，新薬市販直後の安全対策の重要性です。米国では1999年，FDAの報告書（Managing the Risks from Medical Product Use）がその重要性を指摘していました。報告書では，使用新薬については医療機関を限定して販売することや専門医療機関や専門医に限定して販売すること，使用に当たっては一定の教育を受けることなど，市販直後のリスク最小化の導入を提言していました。

日本では1993年のソリブジン事件（第2章参照）を契機として，その後，市販直後の安全対策の重要性が強く認識され，その後，市販直後調査が2001年から導入されました。この制度は，新薬発売の6か月間に，新薬が納入される医療機関すべてに対し，一定の頻度で適正使用の徹底を伝え，重篤な事象があれば速やかに報告するように依頼することを企業に義務付けたものです（詳細は第4章および「日本における医薬品のリスクマネジメント」を参照）。

第2は，世界に先駆けて薬事法に規定した「承認条件」です。この規定は，昭和35（1960）年に薬事法第79条に規定されました（詳細は第4章参照）。開発段階で安全性等に関する情報が特に限られている医薬品や承認後の安全性確保が特に必要な医薬品について，「承認条件」が付与されます。「承認条件」は大きく分けて，①承認後一定期間または一定症例数に達するまで医薬品を使用した患者のすべての情報の収集を義務付けるもの（全例調査），②承認後追加的な臨床試験を義務付けるもの（市販後臨床試験），③承認後一定期間，医薬品を使用できる医療機関または医師を限定（使用限定）するものがあります。

第3は，医薬品副作用被害救済制度です。サリドマイド事件やスモン事件をきっかけとして，医薬品の副作用による被害者の迅速な救済を図ることを目的として導入され，1980年から救済業務が開始されました。医薬品が適正に使用されたにもかかわらず発生した一

restitution. In other words, except in an extremely small number of cases, the liability of healthcare professionals has not been the issue in question. These facts have informed the characteristics of safety measures for drugs and medical devices adopted in Japan. Discussion regarding prevention of recurrence of drug-induced suffering at courts and on other relevant occasions has successfully contributed to reinforcement of the Japanese pharmaceutical regulations in each step from development through to use in the market. On the side of the administration, a system to strictly monitor development stages through to post-marketing and a system involved in approval review and safety measures have been reinforced. In addition, a relief services system for adverse health effect caused by drugs, etc. and a relief system for infections acquired through biological products have been established. Table 2 summarizes how the lessons from the major incidents of drug-induced suffering were linked with changes to the pharmaceutical regulations.

In Japan, on the basis of the policy that continuous and consistent risk management is required for the whole life of a drug from development to post-marketing (life-cycle risk management) in order to secure post-marketing safety of new drugs, a conditional approval system (for which the revised Pharmaceutical Affairs Law (PAL) in 2002 has established penalties) and an early post-marketing phase risk minimization and vigilance (EPRV) system were introduced before North American and European countries. This policy was a driving force behind the development of E2E Guidelines under ICH. In the 1990s, the Japanese pharmaceutical regulatory system with special regards to safety securing measures was a step ahead of that in North American and European countries. Three major characteristics of the Japanese pharmaceutical regulatory system are described below.

First of all, safety securing measures in an early phase after the launch of a new drug are given importance. In 1999 in the US, a FDA's report entitled "Managing the Risks from Medical Product Use" pointed out this importance and proposed introduction of risk minimization actions in the early post-marketing phase, e.g. by initially restricting the number of medical institutions to which a new drug is sold, restricting sales only to specialized medical institutions and specialists, and requiring physicians and other relevant healthcare professionals to undertake predetermined training.

In Japan, the sorivudine incident in 1993 (see Chapter 2) highlighted and made the individuals concerned recognize the importance of risk minimization measures in an early post-marketing phase, which triggered introduction of the EPRV system in 2001. This system requires that for the first 6 months after the start of marketing, marketing authorization holders (MAHs) shall have the obligation to make periodic requests to all medical institutions, to which they deliver their new drugs, so as to fully disseminate information on the proper use of the drug concerned within the medical institution, and to ask them to make a prompt report whenever any serious event should occur (for more detailed information, please see Chapter 4 and refer to the book entitled "Drug Risk

表2 戦後の日本の主な薬害事件と薬事規制への反映

主な薬害事件	整備・強化された薬事規制
サリドマイド事件	・医薬品の製造承認に関する基本方針制定(添付資料の明確化,新開発医薬品の副作用報告等) ・医薬品副作用報告制度(医薬品副作用モニター制度,企業報告制度,薬局モニター制度の創設,国際医薬品モニター制度への参加)の法制化
スモン事件	・薬事法改正(再評価・再審査制度の法制化,企業の副作用報告の義務化,緊急命令・回収命令規定の新設,臨床試験に関する規定の新設(治験依頼の基準,GCP,治験届出制度)等) ・医薬品副作用被害救済基金法制定(医薬品副作用被害救済制度の新設)
ソリブジン事件	・薬事法改正等(治験依頼者の責任強化,医薬品適正使用の導入,添付文書記載要領の見直し,緊急FAX網の導入,企業からの副作用報告期間の短縮等) ・医薬品医療機器審査センター新設(審査体制の強化) ・市販直後調査制度新設(新薬販売開始直後の安全性の確保)
エイズ事件	・薬事法改正等(企業の感染症報告および海外措置報告の義務化,GCPなどの義務化,承認・許可制度の抜本的見直し) ・厚生省の審査・安全対策の強化(危機管理体制の強化,生物由来製品とその他の医薬品の審査・安全性・監視にかかわる部門の連携強化等) ・安全な血液製剤の安定供給の確保等に関する法律改正(生物由来製品の安全性確保の充実,市販後安全対策の強化) ・独立行政法人医薬品医療機器総合機構法制定(感染症被害救済制度の新設,審査・安全対策業務の充実・強化)
薬害肝炎事件	「薬害再発防止のための医薬品行政等の見直しについて(最終提言)」の公表。薬害教育の導入(初等中等教育,高等教育など)。

定以上の健康被害に対して,医療費,障害年金,遺族年金等が支払われます。この制度により,被害者は負担の大きい裁判によらなくとも救済が可能となりました。この制度の適

Table 2 Major post-war drug-induced sufferings in Japan and their impact on the pharmaceutical regulations

Major incidents	Newly established and reinforced pharmaceutical regulations
Thalidomide incident	· Establishment of the "Basic Policy on Approval for Manufacture of Drugs" (including, among others, clarification of data to be submitted with approval applications, and adverse drug reaction (ADR) reporting for newly developed drugs) · Legalization of the ADR reporting systems (newly established systems : an ADR monitoring system, a system under which marketing authorization holders (MAHs) shall report ADRs to the regulatory authorities, and a system to collect information on ADRs from recommended pharmacies; and participation in the International Drug Monitoring Program)
SMON incident	· Revision of the Pharmaceutical Affairs Law (PAL) (including, among others, legalization of the reexamination and reevaluation systems, making it obligatory for MAHs to report ADRs, new establishment of regulations to place orders for emergency measures and for recall, and new establishment of regulations for clinical studies (criteria for sponsoring clinical trials, GCP, a clinical trial notification system)) · Establishment of the "Act on Adverse Drug Reaction Relief Services Fund" (new establishment of the Relief System for Adverse Drug Reactions)
Sorivudine incident	· Revision of the PAL, etc. (including, among others, reinforcement of the responsibilities of sponsors, introduction of the concept of proper use of drugs, review of the guidelines for completing package inserts, introduction of an emergency FAX network, and shortening of the ADR reporting period during which MAHs should make required reports) · New establishment of the Pharmaceutical and Medical Devices Evaluation Center (PMDEC) (in order to reinforce the review system for approval for new drugs) · New establishment of an early post-marketing phase risk minimization and vigilance (EPRV) system (in order to secure the safety of a new drug immediately after its launch onto the market)
AIDS incident	· Revision of the PAL, etc. (making it obligatory for MAHs to report infectious diseases and actions taken overseas, obligation to observe GCP and other relevant regulations, and radical review of the system granting approvals and licenses) · Reinforcement of the Ministry of Health and Welfare's review and safety measures (including, among others, reinforcement of risk management system, and enhancement of collaboration between the functions responsible for biological products and those responsible for other products in terms of review, safety measures, and vigilance) · Revision of the "Law on Securing Stable Supply of Safe Blood Products" (improvement of securing safety of biological products, and reinforcement of post-marketing pharmacovigilance) · Establishment of the "Act on the Pharmaceuticals and Medical Devices Agency" (new establishment of the Relief System for Infections Acquired through Biological Products, and improvement and enhancement of review- and safety-related activities)
Drug-induced hepatitis incident	Announcement of the "Review of the Drug Administration for Preventing Recurrence of Drug-Induced Sufferings (Final Proposal)". Introduction of education regarding drug-induced suffering (at primary, secondary, and higher education, and on other relevant occasions)

Management in Japan").

用は裁判による補償とは独立しています。この制度はエイズ事件など生物由来製品による感染等の健康被害の救済へと発展し，生物由来製品感染症等被害救済制度が2004年に作られました。この制度は次第に，国民および医療関係者に知られるようになりましたが，救済事業を委託されている医薬品医療機器総合機構は，一層その周知に努めています。

　さらに被害の救済という点では，産科医療補償制度もユニークなものです。産科領域における被害の救済にとどまらず，被害の低減，医事紛争の減少につながることが期待されています。

　以上に概括した通り，最近まで，日本は市販後安全対策の制度が最も整備されている国の一つであると国際的にも認められていました。その意味では，日本での薬害による教訓は薬事制度に活かされてきたと言えます。そしてこの制度を活かすためには，導入された背景や契機となった事件を理解した上で，患者の利益と安全性を優先する文化を育てることが不可欠です。

　一方，薬害事件の中には，医療現場での不適正使用によると理解されるものも含まれています。冒頭に述べたように，日本では薬害が刑事裁判になることは極めてまれであり，また民事裁判においては，医療現場の問題は取り上げられることは少ないのです。したがって薬害事件の教訓は，必ずしも医療現場における適正使用の推進に活かされていないと言えます。この問題は，日本における安全対策推進上今後につながる大きな課題であると言えます。

The second characteristic is the conditional approval system specified in the PAL. Japan was an international pioneer in establishing such a system. The provisions regarding conditions for license, accreditation and approval were stipulated in Article 79 of the PAL in 1960 (for more detailed information, please see Chapter 4). The approval conditions are especially given to drugs for which information on safety, etc. obtained in the development phase is limited or post-approval risk minimization measures are particularly required. There are three major conditions as follows: (1) a condition that makes it obligatory to collect information on all patients using the drug for a fixed period after approval or until a certain number of patients is reached (all-patient post-marketing surveillance); (2) a condition that makes it obligatory to perform additional clinical studies after approval (post-marketing clinical study); and (3) a condition that makes it obligatory to restrict use of the drug by limiting the medical institutions or physicians that can access the drug for a fixed period after approval (restricted access).

The third characteristic is the Relief System for Adverse Drug Reactions. The thalidomide incident and the SMON incident triggered establishment of this system with the aim of immediately providing relief to victims of adverse drug reactions (ADRs). Provisions of relief benefits started in 1980. Specifically, medical fees, disability pensions, survivors' pensions, etc. are paid for health damage exceeding a certain level that could not be prevented in spite of proper use of a drug. Because of this system, victims can receive relief benefits without bearing the great burden of going to court. Application of this system is independent from compensation ordered by the court. This system further developed into a relief system for health damage caused by biological products, such as infection, the health damage in the AIDS incident. As a result the Relief System for Infections Acquired through Biological Products was established in 2004. These systems have gradually been recognized by the general public and healthcare professionals, although the Pharmaceuticals and Medical Devices Agency (PMDA) that is entrusted with the relief services is attempting to increase the public's awareness of these systems.

The Japan Obstetric Compensation System for Cerebral Palsy is also unique in terms of victims' relief. It is expected that this system will contribute to reduction of health hazard and medical disputes, in addition to provision of relief to victims in the obstetric field.

As summarized above, until recently it has been recognized internationally that Japan is one of the countries with the best-organized post-marketing safety measures. This fact represents that the lessons from the drug-induced suffering are reflected in the Japanese pharmaceutical regulatory system. For the purpose of making the best use of this system, it is essential to foster a culture prioritizing patients' benefit and safety on the basis of good understanding of the background behind introduction of the system and the incidents triggering its establishment.

2. 薬害事件の分析と考察

1）分析と考察についての留意点

　私たちはこの薬害の事例から将来に向けての知恵を学びたいと思っていますが，その際にいくつかの大事なことに留意しておく必要があります．

　まず，第一に本書で取り上げた15件の事件はたまたま今日まで記録が残り，社会的にも記憶されていたものです．一方，事件にまで発展しなかった事例やあるいは記憶にも留められなかった事件も多数あると思われます．今後は，このような事件の掘り起しと検証も積み重ねる必要があります．

　第二に，事件の客観的な再現は不可能であり，記録の取捨選択や評価者のバイアスが避けられないものです．しかし，日本の薬害の歴史全体を俯瞰した時に見えてくるものを，他国のそれらと比較して考察することで，より妥当な教訓が得られると考えます．日本の事例を各国の事例と比較対照して，洞察を加えていただけることを期待します．

　第三に，薬害は医療文化の産物の一つであることから，その国の社会的状況を抜きにしては語れません．そのため，制度を含め社会状況の異なる他国では，理解しがたいことがあると考えられます．薬害を医薬品にかかわる薬事規制というフレーミングでとらえることは極めて重要ですが，できるだけ幅広い視点で考察することが重要であると考えます．

2）日本人と薬

　2012年，日本の医薬品の売上高は7兆6000億円で世界第2位です．一人当たり61,000円（610ドル：1ドル100円として）の医薬品を使用しているので，日本人は薬好きと言われています．日本の文化的社会的な背景にふれておきたいと思います．

　今日，日本人の多くが日常的に意識しているわけではありませんが，仏教的思考は日本文化の底流の一つです．日本仏教思想には，「病気平癒」という信仰があります．中世の寺院創建の目的の多くは，病気平癒でした．また信仰の対象として薬師如来という仏像があります．"薬師"寺という名称を冠する，薬草を管理した（当時の）国営の寺院も日本各

On the other hand, some of the drug-induced sufferings are caused by improper use of drugs in actual medical practice. As described at the beginning of this Chapter, in Japan incidents of drug-induced suffering extremely rarely bring about criminal lawsuits, and in civil lawsuits, on-site problems in medical institutions become issues of litigation in only a small number of cases. Accordingly, lessons from drug-induced suffering do not always contribute to promotion of proper use in clinical settings. This is a future challenging issue to be tackled in order to promote risk minimization measures in Japan.

2. Analysis and Discussion of Drug-Induced Suffering

1) Matters requiring attention in analysis and discussion

From the drug-induced suffering, we want to gain wisdom with which we will take adequate precautions for the future. When analyzing and discussing the past incidents, there are several important matters we need to pay attention to.

First of all, for the 15 incidents of drug-induced suffering summarized in this book, it is fortunate that records have been maintained up until the present, and the incidents remain in society's collective memory. There may have existed many health damage events which did not develop into drug-induced suffering or those of drug-induced suffering which were not remembered. In the future, we need to uncover and verify such incidents so as to compile information and knowledge.

Secondly, it is impossible to objectively reproduce an incident of drug-induced suffering. It is unavoidable that only some fragments of information are picked up and chosen among records of the incident and that individuals performing evaluation of the incident have exerted to a certain degree some personal bias when evaluating it. Nevertheless, comparing what we see when taking a 'bird's eye' overview of the history of drug-induced suffering in Japan with those overseas may provide reasonable lessons. We therefore expect the reader to compare the Japanese incidents or events against those in his or her own country so as to grasp the nature of them.

Thirdly, since drug-induced suffering is one of the byproducts of medical culture, it cannot be separated from the social circumstances in the country concerned. We may not be able to understand fully the situations surrounding drug-induced suffering in other countries which have different social circumstances including pharmaceutical regulations. Although it is extremely important to capture drug-induced suffering within a frame of pharmaceutical regulations, we attempt to discuss it from a broader viewpoint in so far as possible.

2) Japanese people and medicines

In 2012, the sales of drugs in Japan totaled 7,600 billion Japanese Yen (JPY), which ranks second in

地にあります。薬師とは古来日本における医師を兼ねており，医療と薬は分かちがたい文化を持っていました。現代でも，数十年前までは医者に往診してもらった時の医療費は「薬代」と言い習わさていました。このように，日本には薬を受け入れる社会文化的素地が大きかったのです。

　近代医療制度になってからも医者のパターナリズムと相まって，患者が薬を無批判に受け入れてきた傾向があると指摘されています。たとえば筋短縮症事件では，医師が積極的に注射をしたことが原因ですが，親の注射希望に医師が迎合したことが指摘されています。ソリブジン事件では，発売前から患者の強い期待がありました。同様にイレッサ事件においては医師や患者の間で発売前から強い期待がありました。そしてこの期待は企業の営業姿勢，専門家のコメント，報道，行政措置などによって加速，強化されました。

　もう一つ，健康保険制度の導入と発展は，長期にわたって日本の医薬品の消費に大きな影響を与えてきました。日本の健康保険制度はアクセス性と利便性，平等性に優れたシステムです。この健康保険制度は1961年に国民皆保険制度となりました。当時，被保険者は医療という現物支給に対して1割負担を窓口で支払っていました。現在は財政の問題から原則3割負担となっていますが，今日でも依然として有効な制度であり続けています。

　一方，この保険制度では医療行為や医薬品の価格は保険点数で定められており，医薬分業が進んでいなかった20年ほど前まで，基準による公定価格と製薬企業からの納入価格との差が医療機関の利益になっていました。したがって，医療機関における医薬品の使用は，製薬企業の販促活動に大きく影響されてきました。この薬価差益は，日本の健康保険制度の持っている構造的な特徴でした。筋短縮症事件は，注射薬の薬価差益が注射という医療行為のインセンティブになったとされています。現在，日本の医薬分業率は70％程度に向上し，薬価差益は病院の大きな収入源にはなっていません（日本は以前から原則医薬分業です。しかし例外規定のため，実質的には長い間医薬分業が進みませんでした）。しかし，健康保険制度の利便性が過剰医療の傾向を生み出しているとされています。

the world. This equates to an annual consumption of drugs per person of 61,000 JPY (610 US dollars, based on 100 JPY per US dollar), which supports the perceived stereotype that Japanese people consume a substantially high quantity of medicines. The sociocultural background that underlies this is briefly outlined in this section.

The teachings of Buddhism have cultivated one of the undercurrents of Japanese culture, although many Japanese people are not always conscious of this fact while living their daily modern lives. The Japanese Buddhism doctrine contains a belief of "healing all the sick and the injured". In the Medieval Period in Japan, many temples were built for the purpose of healing diseases and injuries. The "Yakushinyorai (the Buddha of Healing)" is an enshrined statue. Temples named "Yakushi (the Medicine Buddha)" exist throughout Japan. These temples were operated by the state (in the Medieval Period) and were responsible for managing medicinal herbs. In Japan, the profession named "Kusushi" (for which the same two Kanji characters are used as in "Yakushi") were specialists in herbal medicine and traditionally functioned as a physician also, which gave rise to a culture closely linking medical care with drugs. Even in modern times, until a few decades ago, healthcare expenses incurred when a doctor made a house call were customarily referred to as "charge for medicine". As such, Japan possesses substantial sociocultural grounds for accepting medicines.

Even after the introduction of a modern healthcare system, in Japan, it is pointed out that patients tended to accept drugs without due consideration, partly because of medical paternalism under which physicians instruct patients about what to do and the patients normally follow the physicians' advice. For example, the muscle contracture incident was caused by intramuscular injections frequently administered by physicians, although it was also pointed out that physicians went along with the desire of patients' parents to place a high and arguably unfounded value on injections. In the sorivudine incident, patients had raised expectations for the drug even prior to its launch onto the market. In the gefitinib incident also, physicians and patients had a great deal of anticipation for the drug even before the start of its marketing. The expectation was accelerated and intensified by the responsible pharmaceutical companies' behavior of marketing, comments given by specialists, media coverage, and actions taken by the drug administration.

Another matter worth mentioning is that the introduction and development of the National Health Insurance (NHI) Scheme has long had a significant impact on consumption of drugs in Japan. The Japanese NHI Scheme is excellent in accessibility, convenience, and equality. This health insurance program became a universal public insurance system in 1961, under which insured persons and their family members are entitled to receive insured medical treatment at relatively low expenses. An insured person paid 10% of his or her medical expenses at hospital in the past, but this proportion

3. 薬害という医原病についての様相

1）薬害の規模

　日本の薬害事件を直接の被害者数でみるとき，比較的小さな規模のものとしてソリブジン事件の数十名から，筋短縮症事件やスモン事件等の1万人といった幅があります。しかし被害規模の確定は，いずれの事件においても困難です。多くの場合，薬害の規模は明らかになっている数字より少なくとも数倍，あるいはそれ以上の規模であると想像することが妥当であると考えられます。たとえばサリドマイド事件では生存者数は確定していますが，死産，流産などその実態は推定によるほかはありません。筋短縮症事件では，隠れた被害者を含めると10万人以上であろうとする研究者もいます。

2）薬害の深刻さ

　薬害の被害はどれをとっても痛ましく，それぞれの健康被害の深刻さを事件ごとに比較することは適切ではありません。死亡を免れても，被害者は深刻でかつ永続的な健康被害に苦悩することになります。これらの健康被害の多くは原状回復が不可能であるか，もしくは回復がきわめて限定的である疾病や傷害であることが特徴です。このため，被害者が高齢化するに伴い，新たな健康不安に悩まされ，またせっかく得た仕事を体調不良からあきらめていかざるを得ないという人生の問題に直面しています。

of cost sharing is currently 30% as a rule because of the financial problems Japan has faced in recent years. This NHI Scheme is still effective as of today.

On the other hand, this NHI Scheme sets up medical fee points for medical services and drugs, on the basis of which medical fees paid to insurance medical care facilities and insurance medical practitioners as well as prices of drugs and medical devices are determined. Until about 20 years ago at which medical practice was not separated from drug dispensing, differences between purchasing prices by medical institutions and the NHI reimbursement prices constituted profit for medical institutions. The use of drugs at medical institutions therefore was greatly influenced by the sales promotion activities of pharmaceutical companies. The profitability due to drug price discrepancy was a structural feature of the Japanese NHI Scheme. Some researchers point out that in the muscle contracture incident, profits born by drug price discrepancy of injections were incentives to perform the medical practice of injection. At present, the rate of separation between medical practice and drug dispensing has improved and reached about 70%. The price discrepancy is never a substantial resource of income of hospital (note that Japan has long adopted as a rule the policy of separating medical from dispensary practices, although in reality the presence of exceptional rules has hindered its taking root on site). Nevertheless, the convenience of the NHI Scheme may result in a tendency toward overmedication.

3. Features of Drug-Induced Suffering, i.e. An Iatrogenic Disease

1) Scale of drug-induced suffering

Analysis of the drug-induced suffering in Japan by the number of victims reveals great differences from a relatively small scale of incident involving several tens of victims such as the sorivudine incident to a large scale of the ten-thousand-level as noted in the muscle contracture incident and the SMON incident. It is difficult to identify the scale of tragedy in any incident. It may be reasonable to imagine that in many cases, the actual scale of drug-induced suffering would be at least several times greater than the determined figure. For example, in the thalidomide incident, the number of survivors is identified, whereas there is no way but to estimate the reality of stillbirths or miscarriages. For the muscle contracture incident, some researchers claim that the total number of victims including unidentified ones exceeds 100,000.

2) Seriousness of drug-induced suffering

Each and every case of drug-induced suffering is tragic and it is difficult to compare incidents in terms of seriousness of health damage. Even if victims survive, they may experience serious and chronic pain due to health damage. In many such cases with health damage, those affected are unlikely to recover to their original state or even if possible, their recovery is extremely limited. For these reasons, victims face their own life-related challenges that accompany aging; they may suffer

3）薬害の多重性

薬害は被害者本人だけでなく，家族に多大な経済的，精神的，肉体的な負担を強いています。サリドマイド事件や陣痛促進剤事件では胎児の被害にとどまらず，母親が自責の念に苦しみました。MMRワクチン事件では，後遺症のてんかんに苦しむ子供を一生支えていくという負担を背負った両親もいます。

4）薬害に対する不条理さという思い

当財団が毎年主催している薬害教育特別研修講座は，薬害被害者を講師として招いています。被害者の思いの最大のものは「なぜ自分がこのような目に遭わなければならなかったのか？」という不条理さに対する疑問です。これまで，薬害については薬事制度や国，企業の責任，経済的補償などの観点からから議論されてきました。しかし薬害の理不尽さに対する疑問は，被害者自身が発言，発信する以外に議論されることはほとんどなく，あってもそれらの機会はきわめて限られたものでした。被害者は不条理を飲み込んだまま人生を送らなければならない，ということは社会的に理解されていない状況におかれています。

5）被害者とその家族への差別

多くの薬害事件で被害者とその家族への差別が生じています。スモン事件，筋短縮症事件などでは医療関係者でさえ偏見と差別があったとされます。スモン事件では健康被害の苦しさゆえの絶望に加え，伝染性疾患ではないかという疑いから社会的偏見もあって，500名以上の自殺者がでたとされます。これらはもっとも痛ましい薬害の二次被害といえます。

6）薬害についての一過性の記憶

薬害についての社会的関心と記憶は，一般に長く続きません。薬害の原因が判明するまで，あるいは裁判に対してはその時々に社会的関心が強くなりますが，その継続性はありません。大きな理由の一つは，これまで薬害を学校教育や専門教育の中で位置づけてこなかったことが指摘されています。若い世代の中には，世界に衝撃を与えたサリドマイド事件さえ知らない医療関係者がいると言われています。このことは，歴史は教育しなければ風化することが避けられないことを示しています。

7）健康被害と薬との関連性の解明

薬害事件においては，被害と薬の因果関係がすぐに判明しない場合もあります。スモン事件は当初，奇病や伝染性疾患あるいは風土病であるとされ，原因がわかるまでに長期間を要しました。筋短縮症事件では，健康被害そのものの存在が長い間見過ごされてきました。サリドマイドによる奇形発生も，少なくとも日本ではすぐに医薬品との関連性が断定できませんでした。慢性疾患に長期使用する薬剤では，健康被害との関連がすぐに推定で

from anxiety of possible occurrence of new health problems or they may have to give up their hard-earned jobs due to deterioration in health.

3) Multiplicity of drug-induced suffering

Drug-induced suffering imposes a great deal of economic, mental, and physical burden to victims' family members in addition to the victims themselves. In both the thalidomide incident and the labor-inducing drugs incident, tragedy occurred not only in fetuses but also their mothers who seriously suffered from a guilty conscience. In the MMR vaccine incident, parents bear a burden of supporting their children who experience pain from epilepsy, a sequela, for their whole life.

4) Feeling aggrieved against drug-induced suffering

The PMRJ sponsors the Basic Training Course for Drug-Induced Suffering every year and invites victims of drug-induced suffering as lecturers of the Course. The greatest feeling of victims is a question about gross unfairness: "Why did I have to experience such extreme distress without reason?" Drug-induced suffering has so far been discussed from different viewpoints including, among others, the pharmaceutical regulatory system, responsibilities of the national government and the companies concerned, and economic compensation. However, the question of how unreasonable drug-induced suffering is has been raised on only very limited occasions where the victims themselves have an opportunity to voice their opinions, and this has rarely been discussed. The situation where victims have to live their own lives while resentfully accepting the complete unexpectedness and unfairness of their situation is not well understood by society.

5) Discrimination against victims and their family members

Many incidents of drug-induced suffering have caused discrimination against victims and their family members. In the SMON incident and the muscle contracture incident, even healthcare professionals had prejudice and discriminated against victims. In the SMON incident, more than 500 victims committed suicide since they lost hope for the future primarily because the health damage was so painful and in addition, there was a harsh prejudice in society that victims contracted a communicable disease which might be passed on to others. These should be regarded as the most serious indirect, secondary tragedies to drug-induced suffering.

6) Transient memory of drug-induced suffering

Social interest in and memory of drug-induced suffering typically does not last long. Until a cause of drug-induced suffering is identified or while lawsuits are ongoing, social interest sometimes becomes greater if there is a trigger to do so, but it cannot be sustained. One of the major causes of this may be the fact that drug-induced suffering is not clearly positioned in education at school and educational programs designed for professionals. Healthcare professionals in the young generation

きないケースが今後もあり得ると考えられます。

8）繰り返して発生する社会現象または疫病としての薬害

日本の薬害の様相と頻度をみていきますと，それらは単に偶然に発生した不運な事例であり，"いずれは発生を予防できる"という，楽観的な態度を取ることはできません。新しい技術（医薬品，医療機器や治療法）は，新たな恩恵とリスクをもって登場すると考えることが妥当です。現代社会では，新しい技術の受容は，期待される恩恵と考えられる危険性を衡量した選択の結果としてフィードバックを得ながら学習し進歩していきます。しかし，そのフィードバックを十分に得る前に次の選択を迫られる，という状況でもあります。

したがって，健康被害と薬害を完全に予防する手段を講じることは極めて困難です。医薬品についても，ゼロリスクは神話と考えるべきです。考えられるリスク低減の手段とともに，被害拡大を押さえ込む施策とマネジメントが不可欠です。日本では，公衆の健康を繰り返して脅かす薬害という社会現象は，もはや公衆衛生的な問題として研究し，継続的な対策を講じていく必要があるのではないでしょうか。

4. 薬害の原因の多様さ

全国薬害被害者団体連絡協議会のスローガンは，「薬害は薬が原因と思っていませんか？」という問いかけをしています。医薬品は本質的に健康被害を発生させる危険性があることから，薬害は医薬品の善し悪し，あるいは医薬品を規制する観点から議論されてきました。事実，承認審査体制や薬事制度は医薬品の進歩とともに，あるいは後追いの形で整備されてきました。しかし被害者は，医薬品そのものに薬害の責任があるのではなく，

do not even know the thalidomide incident that gave a shock all over the world. History fades with the passage of time unless appropriate education on the history is provided to future generations.

7) Identification of the relationship between health damage and the drug

In some cases of drug-induced suffering, a causal relation between health damage and a particular drug may not be immediately identified. In the SMON incident, there were initially incorrect perceptions that SMON was a bizarre or communicable disease or an endemic disease. It took a long time before the cause was identified. In the muscle contracture incident, the presence of health damage itself was overlooked for a long time. For the deformities caused by thalidomide, at least in Japan, its relation to the drug was not immediately determined. Regarding drugs which are long used for treatment of chronic diseases, their relation to health damage, if any occur in the future, may similarly not be immediately identified.

8) Drug-induced suffering, a repeated social phenomenon or an epidemic

The review of drug-induced suffering in Japan in terms of how the individual incidents developed and how frequently they occurred never makes us draw an overly optimistic conclusion that they were unlucky incidents since they occurred merely by chance and "their occurrences will be prevented sometime in the future". It is reasonable to accept that the debut of a new technology (drug, medical device, or therapy) is always associated with new benefits and risks. In the present days, a new technology is accepted by society through the learning process of feedback and responsive action on risks/benefits. However, new drugs are launched onto the market one after another and we have to make a decision to or not to use a new drug before obtaining feedback of sufficient experience on a prior drug.

It is therefore extremely difficult to take actions so as to completely prevent health damage caused by adverse drug reactions and drug-induced suffering. For drugs, we should consider "zero risk" as an unrealistic aspiration. Measures to minimize possible risks as well as policies and management to suppress expansion of damage are essential. From now on, we should regard drug-induced suffering, a social phenomenon which repeatedly jeopardizes the health of the public, as an issue of public health, and take continuous actions to address the issue and minimize the risks.

4. Diversity of Causes of Drug-Induced Suffering

The Japanese National Liaison Council for Associations of Victims of Drug-Induced Suffering has the following slogan: "Don't you think that drug-induced suffering is caused by drugs?" Due to their nature, drugs are associated with risks of causing health hazard and therefore, drug-induced suffering has been discussed from the perspective of whether a drug is good or bad and from the viewpoint of regulating drugs. In fact, the system of approval review and the pharmaceutical

それを生み出し，使う人間に責任があることを本質的に見抜いています。当初は限定的な健康被害であったものが，薬害へと発展していく過程で何が加速させる要因となったかを整理してみます。

1）患者の期待もしくは需要とそれを加速する因子
　健康被害の拡大は，需要の拡大が関連している場合が多いと言えます。しかしその需要の大きさは，純粋に医学的要求からだけでは決まらない部分があります。ゲフィチニブ事件では治療困難な病状に対して，夢の薬というマスコミを巻き込んだ前評判と，薬価基準収載前でも混合診療を受けることができるという行政上の措置も加わって，患者の期待が大きくなったと言われています。大きな需要が予測され，急激な売り上げが予測されること自体が，すでにリスク管理の対象であると考えるべきでしょう。

　サリドマイド事件，スモン事件などでは安全性を強調した企業の宣伝が行われました。アンプル入り風邪薬事件では高度成長時代を背景として，企業戦士に安易な治療法を提供する宣伝が行われました。これらの事例をふまえて，製薬業界では広告の自主規制が行われることになりました。専門家の意見は都合よく広告に利用されることがある，という認識が医療関係者に必要です。

　筋短縮症では患者の両親の間に注射崇拝の傾向があったとされますが，健康保険制度における注射に対する診療報酬も，注射行為を促進するインセンティブとして働いたとされています。

2）専門家あるいは医学関連学会などの責任
　健康被害の原因究明や被害の拡大防止に果たす専門家の責任は，きわめて大きなものです。筋短縮症事件では，若手医師による自主検診団の活動が大きな役割を果たしましたが，医学関連学会などは対応が鈍く，速やかにその責任を果たし得ませんでした。スモン事件では専門家の間違ったウイルス説が患者を苦しめ，製薬企業に加担して裁判を長期化させました。イレッサ事件では専門家の楽観的な意見広告や記事が，患者の期待を加熱させたとされます。今後は，臨床試験に参加した専門家による論文など社会的影響の大きい行為については，利益相反の明言を含む倫理性が求められます。

3）因果関係解明の優先
　スモン事件，サリドマイド事件など，製薬企業が健康被害と薬の因果関係究明を優先したことで，予防措置の実行を先送りした結果として被害を拡大してしまったケースがあります。因果関係を求める姿勢と，行政や企業の組織防衛反応が協働したと考えられます。薬害肝炎に関する提言が「予防原則に立つ」ことを求めているのは，何を優先事項とするか，という問いかけに他なりません。

regulatory system have been improved along with or following advancement of drugs. However, victims have seen through to the truth of drug-induced suffering, i.e. what causes it is not the drugs themselves but those who give birth to and use them. This section focuses on factors which accelerate the process of development from an initially limited scale of health damage to an incident of drug-induced suffering.

1) Patients' expectation or demand and factors accelerating it

Expansion of health damage caused by adverse drug reactions is largely related to increase of demand for the drug concerned. The scale of this demand is not always determined by purely medical requirement. In the gefitinib incident, patients' expectations for this new drug were ballooned unrealistically by the pre-launch talk of "a dream drug" for a disease difficult to treat that received prominent coverage in the mass media since the indication of this drug is difficult to treat, in combination with the administrative decision to permit application of the mixed treatment (note that the mixed treatment means combining medical treatments that are covered by health insurance with treatments that are not) to gefitinib even before its inclusion in the NHI Drug Price List. We should consider that the expectation of great demand for a drug, leading to a forecast of rapid sales increase, is already the subject of risk management.

In the thalidomide incident and the SMON incident, the companies concerned publicized the drugs emphasizing that they were safe. In the cold-medicines-in-ampoules incident, advertisements for providing easygoing remedies were targeted to so-called "corporate warriors" who were exceptionally dedicated and hard-working employees and thus sustained Japan's rapid economic growth. The lessons from these incidents encouraged the pharmaceutical industry to undertake voluntary restraints on advertisement and publicity. Healthcare professionals should be aware that a company may take advantage of experts' opinions when advertising its products so that the advertisement is beneficial to the company, and not necessarily in the interest of the public.

In the muscle contracture incident, it is pointed out that patients' parents tended to lean toward an arguably unfounded reverence for injections, and at the same time medical fees paid for injections under the NHI Scheme functioned as an incentive to promote the medical practice of injection.

2) Responsibilities of specialists or medical associations

Specialists take substantially large responsibilities for exploring causes of health damage and preventing its expansion. In the muscle contracture incident, a voluntary medical checkup group consisting of young physicians played important roles in attempting to explore the cause, whereas medical associations were slow to take responsive actions and thus did not promptly fulfill their responsibilities. In the SMON incident, the incorrect virus-causing theory raised by specialists

4）医療現場における不適正使用

筋短縮症事件の被害者の多くは，医療現場で治療上不必要な筋肉注射の乱用によって引き起こされました。しかし学会などからの警告や指導が適切に行われなかったことが，実地医家における注射乱用に歯止めがかからなかった理由でもありました。陣痛促進剤事件では，添付文書の整備や危険性についての啓発が進んで事態は改善されましたが，それにもかかわらず今なお，陣痛促進剤の使用に関するガイドラインが遵守されずに分娩時の医療事故例が報告されています。産科領域においては裁判となるリスクが他の診療科の4倍にもなるという事実と併せ，産科の医療現場の難しさとともに医療関係者にも問題があることを示唆しています。

5）回収の遅れと不徹底

原因薬剤と目される製品の回収が遅れ，それが不徹底となれば被害拡大につながることは自明です．なぜか回収が不徹底であった例は，サリドマイド事件，エイズ事件です。反対に薬害ではあったものの，原因と疑われた製品が販売中止など，タイムリーな回収措置が取られて被害が速やかに収束した事例もあります。ダイアライザー事件，ソリブジン事件，スモン事件，ウシ心嚢膜による抗酸菌様感染事件などです。回収は企業にとって損失をもたらすため，原因が確定するまでは回収を逡巡する傾向があります。しかし当該製品がもし薬害の原因であった場合，回収の遅れは企業と社会にとって致命的な損失をもたらします。被害拡大防止と同時に企業防衛のリスク管理として，回収を明確に位置づけることが必要であると思われます。

6）情報活用の未熟さ

特に海外情報の共有，あるいは活用が適切に行われなかったことが被害を拡大した事例としては，ペニシリンショック事件，サリドマイド事件，スモン事件，筋短縮症事件，CJD，エイズ事件など多くあります。この問題は行政だけに限らず，企業，学会などにも当てはまります。ソリブジン事件においては，審査段階で重要な海外情報を見落としたまま承認されたことが市販後の安全対策を左右しました。

7）行政権限の適切な行使

行政が販売停止や製品回収の権限を法的に持つようになったのは，スモン事件がきっかけとなりました。その後に起きた薬害事件のいくつかでは速やかに権限が行使され，薬害の拡大が抑えられました。しかしエイズ事件では，被告企業が裁判で「回収が遅れたのは国が命令をださなかったからだ」という主張を行いました。

ゲフィチニブ事件は添付文書の記載の妥当性が裁判で争われました。ゲフィチニブは最初期の分子標的抗がん剤のひとつであり，世界で最初に日本で承認されました。患者の期待と自宅で手軽に服用できる経口剤ということなどから見れば，慎重に市場に送り出す方

caused substantial distress to patients and worked in favor of the defendant company, making the trials continue for an unnecessarily protracted time. In the gefitinib incident, specialists' optimistic issue-advocacy advertisement and articles further raised patients' expectations. In the future, publication of research reports by specialists who participate in clinical studies or other behaviors having a great social impact will require control under strict ethics including clear declaration of conflict of interest.

3) Priority given to identification of causality

In the SMON incident and the thalidomide incident as well as other cases, the pharmaceutical companies concerned gave priority to exploration of a causal relation between health damage and drugs and thus put off implementing preventive measures, resulting in expansion of health damage. This may be explained by collaboration of the companies' desire to identify causality with the defensive action to protect an organization that the companies and the regulatory authorities had. The Proposal issued on the drug-induced hepatitis requires the necessity of "standing on precautionary principle", and this is nothing short of constantly asking ourselves the question: "What should be given priority?"

4) Improper use in clinical settings

In the muscle contracture incident, many of the victims were involved due to abuse of intramuscular injections at medical practice sites which were administered at unnecessarily high frequencies for treatment. The relevant scientific associations did not give adequate warning or guidance and this did not put a brake on the abuse of general practitioners providing too many injections. In the labor-inducing drugs incident, repeated revisions of package inserts and dissemination of information on risks have greatly improved the situation. Still now, however, there are reports of medical accidents upon delivery due to noncompliance with the guidelines on the use of labor-inducing drugs, which indicates, together with the fact that a risk of bringing about lawsuits is as high as 4 times greater in the obstetric field than in other medical fields, how difficult it is to manage medical practice and healthcare professionals may be more prone to inadequate practice in this field.

5) Delay and inadequacy in recall

It is self-evident that if recall of a causative drug is delayed and in addition, not well executed, it will cause health damage to expand. In the thalidomide incident and the AIDS incident, recalls were performed inadequately for unknown reasons. In contrast, in the dialyzer induced ophthalmologic disorders incident, the sorivudine incident, the SMON incident, and the incident of bovine pericardium induced infection with probably acid-fast bacilli, adequate recall actions were taken in a timely manner, e.g. sales of the products that were suspected to have caused health damage were promptly discontinued, and the health damage came to an end soon afterwards. Notwithstanding,

策が必要でした。そのためには，全例調査という承認条件を付け，重篤な副作用発生後は被害の拡大を防ぐため，すみやかに緊急安全性情報の発出を指示すべきだったという意見が強くあります。

　これらの事例は法的に権限が整備されていても，適切に行使することが行政にとっての重要課題であることを示しています。

8)関係者間におけるリスクコミュニケーション
　多くの薬害事件で，行政組織内部，行政組織と企業，学会間，企業と医療従事者など様々な関係者間のコミュニケーションが不良であったことを，被害拡大の要因として指摘することができます。発売後，医療従事者には主に企業からの情報が提供されますが，審査報告書の内容を発売に合わせて公表することによって，医療関係者に公平な判断の機会を与えることもコミュニケーションの一助として考えられます。

these latter incidents still comprised drug-induced suffering, but their impacts were limited due to the prompt response. Since recall results in financial losses on companies, they tend to hesitate in recalling their products until a cause is identified. However, if the product concerned is a cause of drug-induced suffering, then delayed recall of that product causes fatal losses to both the company concerned and society. It is therefore necessary to take actions to prevent expansion of health damage and at the same time, to clearly position recall within a company's defensive risk management framework.

6) Immature utilization of information

In many cases including the penicillin shock incident, the thalidomide incident, the SMON incident, the muscle contracture incident, the CJD incident, and the AIDS incident, inadequacy in sharing or utilization of overseas information in particular caused expansion of damage. This problem is applied to not only the regulatory authorities but also companies and scientific associations. In the sorivudine incident, the facts that the important overseas information was overlooked during the stage of review for approval and the drug was approved had influence on the post-marketing safety measures.

7) Proper use of administrative authority

In Japan, the administration did not have legal power to order discontinuation of marketing or recall of products until the SMON incident. In some of the subsequent incidents of drug-induced suffering, the administration promptly used its power to suppress expansion of drug-induced suffering. In the AIDS incident, however, the defendant company claimed in the litigation that "the recall was delayed because the national government did not issue an order of recall".

In the gefitinib incident, the appropriateness of what was stated in the package insert was the focal point of the trial. Considering the facts that gefitinib was one of the earliest molecularly targeted anticancer agents that was approved in Japan first in the world, and that patients had great expectations for the drug and due to its oral formulation, easily took it at home, actions should have been taken to make the company cautious in launching the drug onto the market. For this purpose, there is a strong opinion that all-patient post-marketing surveillance should have been attached to the drug as a condition for approval and that after the occurrences of serious adverse drug reactions, issuance of an Urgent Safety Information should immediately have been instructed in order to prevent the expansion of health damage.

These incidents indicate that even though the legal power is established, what is most important for the administration is to use it properly.

5. 薬害裁判

　日本では多くの薬害が訴訟となりました。ジフテリア予防接種事件は刑事裁判となり，エイズ事件は刑事裁判と民事裁判が行われました。一方，スモン事件，サリドマイド事件，C型肝炎事件，陣痛促進剤事件，ゲフィチニブ事件は民事裁判となりました。そしてすべてが長期の裁判の後に，和解で決着しています（ゲフィチニブ事件は2013年4月に原告敗訴の最高裁判決）。総じて提訴から決着までの期間は10年以上であり，最長は筋短縮症事件の18年間でした。和解金額は一般に賠償請求額に比べて大幅に低くなっています。

　日本の裁判においては，原告がカルテなどの保全を行わなくてはならないため，医師を被告とするケースはほとんどありません。そのため，薬害裁判の多くは国，製薬企業を被告としています。国や製薬企業に比べて患者の立場は経済力，情報リテラシーなどあらゆる面において非力であることが，裁判あるいは和解における非対称な力関係を生んでいるといえます。原告は長期の裁判に疲弊し，不満足であっても和解を選択せざるを得なくなっています。日本の薬害事件の裁判が和解で決着することの理由の一つが，原告と被告の非対称性にあると考えられます。

　不条理な被害を余儀なくされた被害者とその家族が，原状回復のために長期の人生を費やして裁判を闘わなければならないこと，結果として不十分な金額で決着せざるを得ないことは，薬害のもたらすもう一つの加害性と言うべきでしょう。回復が困難な健康被害を被った被害者は，加齢に伴う健康状態の低下と日常生活の制約が次第に顕著になってきています。薬害の被害を一時的な和解金で解決することの限界が，数十年を経て明らかになってきています。

　ゲフィチニブ事件は，製造販売企業の添付文書記載の妥当性を巡って争われました。要点は，問題となった間質性肺炎に関する記載が，使用上の注意の上から4番目であり，警告性が不十分であったというものです。つまり添付文書という製造物責任に関するものでした。しかしすでに2章で見てきたように，ゲフィチニブ事件も多くの要素が絡んで発生したものです。各国の法体系の違いから他国の裁判と同列に考えることはできませんが，

8) Risk communication among the individuals concerned

In many incidents of drug-induced suffering, a factor leading to expansion of health damage was poor communication among a variety of stakeholders including, among others, functions inside the administrative organizations, between the administrative bodies and companies, among scientific associations, and between companies and healthcare professionals. After a new drug is launched onto the market, the relevant information is provided primarily by its MAH(s) to healthcare professionals. Publication of the contents of a documented review report on a new drug at the time of its launch onto the market may improve communication since such publication would give opportunities of making an unbiased decision to healthcare professionals.

5. Drug-Induced Suffering Litigation

In Japan, many incidents of drug-induced suffering brought about lawsuits: criminal lawsuits in the diphtheria immunization incident; both criminal and civil lawsuits in the AIDS incident; and civil lawsuits in the SMON incident, the thalidomide incident, the hepatitis C virus infection incident, the labor-inducing drugs incident, and the gefitinib incident. All court cases continued over a long time and were eventually settled (note that in the gefitinib incident, the Supreme Court issued a judgment against the plaintiff in April 2013). Overall, it took over 10 years from the time of filing lawsuits to the conclusion of litigation. The longest was 18 years for the muscle contracture incident. Generally, the amount of settlement was substantially lower than the amount of damages claimed.

In Japanese civil cases, since the plaintiff has to preserve medical records or other relevant evidence, medical doctors are rarely defendants. For this reason, lawsuits regarding drug-induced suffering are filed in many cases against the national government and pharmaceutical companies as defendants. Patients are much weaker in power than the national government and pharmaceutical companies in every aspect including, among others, economic power and information literacy, which produces an imparity between the plaintiff and the defendant in litigation or settlement. The plaintiff is exhausted by long-lasting trials and feels that there is nothing but to accept settlement even if they are not satisfied with it. One of the reasons why cases of drug-induced suffering in Japan are settled may be the imparity between plaintiff and defendant.

Victims of drug-induced suffering are forced to suffer from significantly unjust health damage against their will. These victims and their family members have to spend a substantial part of their lives to fight in court so as to seek personal restitution, and as a minimum have to accept an insufficient amount of settlement to conclude their cases. This reality should be regarded as another injury-inflicting aspect of drug-induced suffering. Victims who suffer from health damage which is difficult to recover are clearly aware that their health condition is deteriorated by aging, putting more restrictions on their daily living activities. Several tens of years after the settlement, it becomes

添付文書に関する製造物責任という争点で薬害裁判を闘うには限界があったことを示しました。

6．まとめ

　日本の薬害事例を通してみるとき，この数十年間で制度的にも概念的にも医薬品の安全確保に関する進歩が見られました。同時に，薬事規制の強化だけでは，薬害発生の予防や被害拡大の最小化に限界があると考えられます。

　薬が本質的に危険性をはらんでいることは医療関係者であれば誰しも理解していることですが，それが広範な社会現象となるときには，社会，文化，医療ニーズ，医療技術など，多様な要素が複合的に絡み合っていることが分かります。しかしある薬害事件でどの要素が重要な役割を果たしたか，ということはそれぞれのケースで異なります。また，社会現象の常として，原因と結果が必ず対になっているとは限らないのです。

　しかし，薬による限定的な健康被害が薬害に拡大するまでに，複合的要素のどれかが適切に機能していれば，事態は大きく変わっていたと思われる事例が多くみられます。したがって，承認の段階で適切な審査を尽くすとともに，市販後の安全対策のためには，市販後のリスク要因の分析とモニタリングが不可欠と考えられます。そして，被害拡大の兆候を検出したときには，因果関係の確定を待つことなく措置を講じることができれば，限りなく薬害発生の未然防止に近づいていくといえるでしょう。

　日本の薬害事例を概括するとき，薬害発生の予防と被害最小化を公衆衛生の課題と位置づけることが，薬事行政と，公共財である医薬品を事業とする企業，そして医療従事者にとって重要であると考えます。

evident that the settlement of drug-induced suffering cases with one-off payment has limitations and may likely be insufficient.

In the gefitinib incident, the focal point of the trial was the appropriateness of what was stated in the package insert prepared by the MAH. The plaintiff claimed that the adverse drug reaction concerned, i.e. interstitial pneumonia, was listed fourth from the top on the list of clinically significant adverse reactions in the section of "Precautions" and therefore, the MAH did not sufficiently warn against it. In other words, the trial's issue was related to product liability for a package insert. As described in Chapter 2, however, many factors became involved in the occurrence of the gefitinib incident, as in the other cases. This case demonstrates that filing a product liability lawsuit alleging defective package insert in drug-induced suffering had limitations, although we cannot compare Japanese court cases with overseas ones in the same terms since each country has its own legal framework.

6. Summary

Overview of drug-induced suffering in Japan underlines the advancement in securing drug safety for the last several ten years from the viewpoints of both systems and concepts. At the same time, only reinforcement of the pharmaceutical regulations has limitations in terms of prevention of occurrence of drug-induced suffering and minimization of health damage expansion.

Every healthcare professional understands that due to their very nature, drugs carry risks. When the danger of a risk develops into a widespread social phenomenon, diverse factors, such as society, culture, medical care need, medical care technology, and other relevant ones, provide added complexity in such development. Which factors play important roles in an incident of drug-induced suffering differs case by case. In addition, a cause is not always paired with a result, which is the way of the social phenomenon.

Evaluation of how an initially limited health damage caused by a drug developed into an incident of drug-induced suffering has demonstrated that in many of the incidents, if any of the factors involved had functioned properly, a greatly different situation might have resulted. It is therefore essential to make every effort to perform an adequate review at the stage of approval. For securing safety in the post-marketing phase, it is inevitable to analyze and monitor post-marketing risk factors. If a sign of damage expansion is detected, responsive actions should be adequately taken without waiting for the identification of causality. These actions may bring us closer to the realization of preventing occurrence of drug-induced suffering.

When summarizing the incidents of drug-induced suffering in Japan, it is important for the drug

administration, companies handling drugs, i.e. the public property, as business, and healthcare professionals to position prevention of drug-induced suffering and damage minimization as issues of public health.

chapter 4

参考資料

REFERENCE DATA

1　薬害再発防止のための医薬品行政の見直しについての概要
2　緊急安全性情報(イエローレター)と発出の実績
3　医薬品リスク管理計画指針について
4　医薬品リスク管理計画の策定について
5　薬害に関する公的教育について
6　全国薬害被害者団体連絡協議会
7　承認条件
8　市販直後調査制度
9　医薬品副作用被害救済制度の概要
10　PMDAの理念
11　日本の薬害年表

1　Summary of the Review of the Drug Administration for Preventing Recurrence of Drug-induced Sufferings
2　Previously Issued Urgent Safety Information (Yellow Letter)
3　Risk Management Plan Guidance
4　Development of Risk Management Plan
5　Public Education of Drug-Induced Suffering
6　Japanese National Liaison Council for Associations of Victims of Drug-Induced Suffering
7　Conditional Approval System
8　Early Post-marketing Phase Risk Minimization and Vigilance (EPRV) system
9　Summary of the Relief Service for Adverse Drug Reactions
10　Our philosophy (PMDA)
11　Chronological Table of Drug-Induced Suffering in Japan

薬害再発防止のための医薬品行政の見直しについての概要

〈最終提言〉

— 2010年4月28日 —

薬害肝炎事件の検証及び再発防止のための医薬品行政のあり方検討委員会
厚生労働省医薬食品局

Ⅰ．はじめに

○ 本委員会は，薬害肝炎事件を検証し再発防止のための医薬品行政の見直しを提言することを目的に設置した。

○ 開催経過：2008年5月から2010年3月までの間に23回開催した。

Ⅱ．薬害肝炎事件の経過から抽出される問題点

○ 薬害肝炎事件の経過の中から，今後の再発防止という観点から抽出される問題点を整理した。
 (1) フィブリノゲン製剤に関する経過関連
 (2) 第Ⅸ因子製剤に関する経過関連
 (3) 上記製剤を通じた事実関係

○ 2009年度には新たに以下の検証を実施し，問題点を整理した。
 (1) 事件当時の行政及び製薬企業の担当者へのヒアリング
 (2) 医療関係者の意識調査(医師を対象としたアンケートやインタビュー)
 (3) 被害者の実態調査(患者及び遺族の調査)

Ⅲ．これまでの主な医薬品行政制度改正の経過

○ 医薬品行政のこれまでの主な制度改正を整理した。
○ 薬事法改正に関する経過関係
○ 医薬品行政組織に関する変遷関係

Ⅳ．薬害防止のための医薬品行政の見直し(詳細については別紙参照)

○ 薬害の再発防止のための医薬品行政の抜本的見直しを提言した。
 (1) 基本的な考え方
  ①医薬品行政に携わる者に求められる基本精神と，薬事法の見直し
  ②医薬品行政に関する行政機関の体制改善と，その行政に携わる人材の育成
  ③薬害と医薬品評価についての教育
  ④「薬害研究資料館」の設立

Summary of the Review of the Drug Administration for Preventing Recurrence of Drug-induced Sufferings
⟨ Final Proposal ⟩
— April 28, 2010 —

Examination committee on verification of the drug-induced hepatitis events and on the desirable drug administration for prevention of its recurrence

Pharmaceutical and Food Safety Bureau, Ministry of Health, Labour and Welfare

I. Introduction

○ The committee was set up for the purpose of verifying the drug-induced hepatitis events and proposing reviews of the drug administration for prevention of its recurrence.

○ Committees : held 23 times from May, 2008 to March, 2010

II. Problems that are extracted from the process of the drug-induced hepatitis events

○ From the process of the drug-induced hepatitis events, problems extracted from the viewpoint of prevention of future recurrence were sorted out.
   (1) On the process related to fibrinogen preparation
   (2) On the process related to factor IX preparation
   (3) Facts through the above preparations

○ Based on the new following verifications implemented in FY2009, the problems were sorted out.
   (1) Hearings from persons in charge in the administration and the drug companies at the time of the events occurred
   (2) Consciousness survey of healthcare providers (Questionnaire of and/or interview with doctors)
   (3) Fact-finding survey of the sufferers (Investigation of the patients and the bereaved)

III. Progress of the main system revisions of drug administration up to now

○ Past main system revisions of the drug administration were marshaled.

○ Regarding progress related to the revision of the Pharmaceutical Affairs Law (PAL)

○ Regarding changes related to the organization of the drug administration

IV. Review of drug administration for preventing drug-induced sufferings(for details, please refer to Appendix)

○ Fundamental review of drug administration for preventing recurrence of drug-induced sufferings was proposed.
   (1) Basic viewpoint
       i) Basic spirit required for people who are involved in drug administration, and review of PAL
       ii) Improving governmental system related to the drug administration, and fostering the human

　　　　　⑤薬剤疫学の専門家の育成と，薬剤疫学分野における研究等の推進
　(2) 臨床試験・治験
　(3) 承認審査
　　　　　①安全性・有効性の評価
　　　　　②審査手順，審議の中立性・透明性
　　　　　③添付文書
　　　　　④再評価
　(4) 製造販売後リスク管理(安全対策)
　　　　　①情報収集体制の強化
　　　　　②収集された／得られた情報の評価(新たなリスク管理手法の導入)
　　　　　③リスクコミュニケーション(リスクに関する情報提供)向上のための情報の積極的かつ円滑な提供と患者・消費者の関与
　　　　　④副作用情報の被害者自身への伝達と，望ましい情報開示
　　　　　⑤適正な情報提供及び広告による医薬品の適正使用
　　　　　⑥GMP査察
　　　　　⑦GVP，GQP査察
　　　　　⑧個人輸入
　(5) 医療機関におけるリスク管理(安全対策)
　(6) 健康被害救済制度
　(7) 専門的な知見を有効に活用するための方策
　(8) 製薬企業に求められる基本精神等

V．医薬品行政を担う組織の今後の在り方(詳細については別紙参照)

○ 医薬品行政の組織についての議論を整理した。
　・医薬品行政組織の一元化(国か独立法人か)などの論点が主として議論された。2009年度に，職員に対するアンケート調査を実施した。
　・最終的には国が責任を負う形にすることなど，組織の形態にかかわらず，医薬品行政組織の望ましい在り方を指摘した。
○ 第三者監視・評価組織の創設
　・薬害の発生及び拡大を未然に防止するため，医薬品行政に関わる行政機関の監視及び評価を行い，適切な措置を採るよう提言を行う「第三者組織」を設置する必要がある。

resources involved
- iii) Education of drug-induced sufferings and of drug evaluation
- iv) Establishment of "the drug-induced sufferings research and resource center"
- v) Fostering the experts in pharmacoepidemiology and promoting studies etc. in the area

(2) Clinical trials

(3) Approval reviews
- i) Evaluation of safety and efficacy
- ii) Review procedure, neutrality and transparency of its deliberation
- iii) Package insert
- iv) Re-evaluation

(4) Post-marketing risk management (safety measures)
- i) Reinforcement of the system for collecting information
- ii) Evaluation of the collected/obtained information (introduction of new risk management method)
- iii) Active and smooth provision of the information and involvement of patients and consumers for improvement of risk communication
- iv) Communication of adverse reaction information to the sufferer him/herself and desirable information disclosure
- v) Proper drug use by appropriate communication of information and advertisement
- vi) GMP inspection
- vii) GVP, GQP inspections
- viii) Personal import

(5) Risk management (Safety measures) in medical institutions

(6) Adverse health effects relief system

(7) Policy to utilize professional knowledge effectively

(8) Basic spirit etc. required for drug companies

V. Desirable structure of the organization bearing drug administration in the future (for details, please refer to Appendix)

○ Discussion about the organization of drug administration was marshaled.
- Mainly issues such as unification of the drug administrative organization (government or an independent administrative agency) were discussed. In FY2009, questionnaire survey of the staffs was conducted.
- Regardless of the form of the organization, the desirable drug administrative organization was pointed out, including that the government has to take final responsibility.

○ Foundation of a third-party monitoring and evaluation body
- To prevent an occurrence of drug-induced suffering and its expansion, it is necessary to establish "a third-party body" which monitors and evaluates the organizations being drug administration, and makes proposals to take appropriate actions.

VI. おわりに

○ 本提言を実現するため，医薬品行政に関する総合的な基本法の制定を検討する必要があるとの意見があった。これも考慮すべきである。

> [注記]
> 日本では，1980年代後半より，フィブリノゲン製剤などの血液製剤によるC型肝炎（当時は非A非B型肝炎と呼ばれていた）ウイルス感染が妊婦を含む患者において報告された。他の製品も含めて，当該製薬企業と国を相手取って訴訟が起こされ，ついには薬害肝炎被害者を救済するための法律が2008年に制定され，原告と厚生労働省は基本合意に達した。この基本合意とその後の議論に基づき，薬害肝炎事件を検証し，その再発防止策のための医薬品行政の在り方を検討するための委員会が設置された。本文書は，最終提言の要約をPMRJ（医薬品医療機器レギュラトリーサイエンス財団）が翻訳したものである。

別紙

IV. 薬害再発防止のための医薬品行政の見直し（概要）

(1) 基本的な考え方
- 医薬品行政の本来の使命は国民の生命と健康を守ることであり，予防原則に立脚した迅速な意志決定が不可欠である。
- 医薬品行政に携わる者及び医療関係者が薬害再発防止のための責務を薬事法に明記すべきである。
- 予防原則に立脚した組織文化の形成のため，国民の生命及び健康を最優先にするとの立場に立った上で，将来にわたる人材を育成しかつ組織とその活動の透明性を確保するための体制を構築
- 承認審査とリスク管理に関わる医薬品行政の体制には，業務量に見合った人員の確保と適切な配置が必要である。
- 医学・薬学等の専門性，高い倫理観，医療現場に対する深い理解といった資質を備える人材の育成及び研修のための対策の検討，ならびに，このような人材が能力を発揮できる環境の確保
- 地方自治体を含む医薬品行政の体制の強化
- 厚生労働省・総合機構と関係分野の人材交流や就業制限を常に検討し，必要な見直しを行うべきである。ただし，製薬企業出身者の就業制限については慎重に検討し対応すべきである。
- 薬害問題や医薬品の評価についての専門教育のみならず，初等中等教育や消費者教育の観点からの生涯教育として薬害を学ぶことについても検討する必要がある。
- 社会の認識を幅広く高めるため，薬害に関する情報の収集や公開を恒常的に行う仕組み（いわゆる薬害研究資料館）を設立
- 薬剤疫学研究を推進するための専門家の養成と公的基金の創設

(2) 臨床試験・治験
- GCP調査の厳格化，臨床試験・治験の被験者の権利保護ならびに健康被害の救済，

VI. Epilogue

○ To realize this proposal, there were opinions that it was necessary to consider the enactment of a general basic law regarding drug administration, and this should also be considered.

> [Note]
> In Japan, infection of Hepatitis C (then, Non-A non-B) virus through the blood products such as fibrinogen preparations was reported among patients including a group of pregnant women from late 1980's. Including other products, lawsuits were raised against the manufacturing companies involved and the government, and eventually Law for the relief of drug-induced hepatitis patients was enacted in 2008 and the plaintiffs reached the basic agreement with the Minister of Health, Labour and Welfare. Based on this agreement and further discussion, a committee was set up in order to verify the drug-induced hepatitis events and to investigate the desirable drug administration for prevention of its recurrence. The above is the translation by PMRJ (Pharmaceutical and Medical Device Regulatory Science Society of Japan) of the summary of the final proposal.

Appendix

IV. Review of drug administration for preventing recurrence of drug-induced sufferings (Summary)

(1) Basic viewpoint

- The original mission of the drug administration is to protect life and health of the nation, and the speedy decision making based on precautionary principle is essential.
- Duties of the people involved in the drug administration as well as healthcare professionals to prevent recurrence of drug-induced sufferings should be specified in PAL.
- Establishing the system to foster human resources for the future and to secure the transparency of the organizations and their activities, giving the top priority to the lives and health of the nation, in order to form an organizational culture based on precautionary principle
- Ensuring staff numbers which meet the quantity of duties and their appropriate placement are necessary for the system of drug administration involved in approval reviews and risk management.
- Considering measures to foster and train human resources qualified with the specialties in medicine or pharmaceutical sciences etc., high ethical standards, and good understanding of medical practices, and ensuring the environment where such human resources can show their abilities
- Reinforcing the system of drug administration including that of local governments
- Personnel exchange and employment restriction among Ministry of Health, Labour and Welfare (MHLW), Pharmaceuticals and Medical Devices Agency (PMDA) and relevant areas should always be examined and these issues should be revisited as needed. However, the employment restriction of persons from drug companies should be carefully reviewed and handled.
- Consideration is needed on not only the professional education about drug-induced sufferings and the evaluation of drugs, but also learning drug-induced sufferings as lifelong learning from the viewpoint of elementary, secondary and consumer education.
- Establishing the arrangement to conduct collection and exhibition of information regarding drug-induced sufferings permanently (so-called "drug-induced sufferings research and

臨床研究が倫理的に問題なく実施できる制度の整備（臨床研究を対象とした法制度で治験との整合性のあるものを整備することを視野に入れた検討を継続して行う），臨床研究に関する情報の登録の義務付けや登録内容と開示範囲の一層の拡大，政府による臨床研究に対する財政支援とそのための公的基金の創設の検討，臨床研究における研究者の権利保護，治験責任医師や試験実施者のあるべき姿の提示と厚生労働省・総合機構による積極的な指導等

(3) 承認審査
- 審査員の資質の向上，承認条件を付すに当たっての指示内容の公表，精査した承認条件に基づく調査結果の速やかな提出と提出された情報の評価の公表
- 審査に係わる審議会（薬事・食品衛生審議会(PFSC)）の審議を公開し，より積極的な開示手続きを通常の審査過程に組み込むことにより，承認審査の透明性を確保
- 医療上の必要性が高くエビデンスのある医薬品が迅速に承認されるよう，総合機構の審査終了から厚生労働省での手続きに要する期間の短縮を考慮
- 添付文書については，最新の知見を適時かつ定期的に添付文書に反映し，添付文書の変更については規制当局と事前に確認し，公的な文書としての位置付けを行い，行政の責任を明確化し，エビデンスに基づく有効性（効能効果）の範囲を科学的に明確にする。
- 不適切な適応外使用が薬害を引き起こしたという教訓を踏まえ，医薬品の適応外使用は，エビデンスに基づき，患者の同意のもとで，真に患者の利益が確保される場合にのみ行うべきである。
- 製薬企業，国，学会は，必要な適応外使用が承認されるよう積極的な役割を果たすべきである。さらに，医療上の必要性が高いものに係わる臨床試験への経済的支援を行うべきである。
- 再評価制度の見直しについては，製薬企業の反証期間に期限を設定し，最新の科学的知見に基づいて添付文書の内容が定期的に見直されるような制度を構築する。

(4) 製造販売後リスク管理（安全対策）
- 医療機関からの副作用報告等の推進，患者からの副作用情報を活用する仕組みの創設，外国規制当局への駐在職員の派遣等の国際連携の強化，国際的な副作用報告データの標準化，将来的に医療現場における様々な安全性情報を一元的に収集・評価し，リスク管理活動に結びつける体制
- 医学・薬学・学剤疫学・生物統計の専門職からなる薬効群ごとのチームが承認審査時と製造販売後に収集された安全性情報を一貫して分析・評価する体制の構築，データマイニングの実装化，ファーマコゲノミクスの調査及び研究の推進
- 予防原則に基づく因果関係の確定前における安全性情報の公表と，そのためのリスク管理体制の構築
- 企業に対して，承認審査の段階から，製造販売後のリスク管理の重点事項や管理手順を定めた計画を提出することを求め，承認後はその計画を適切に実施することを求める「リスク最小化計画実施制度」（仮称）の導入。さらに，ICH-E2Eガイドライ

resource center") to raise social awareness widely
- Training experts and establishing a public fund to promote pharmacoepidemiologic studies

(2) Clinical trials
- More strict GCP examination, protection of rights of the subjects in clinical trials or clinical studies and relief of their health damages, and promotion of the system in which clinical research can be conducted without ethical problem (the consideration will be continued by putting the establishment of legal system covering clinical research consistent with clinical trial in perspective), requirement of registration of the information regarding clinical research and further expansion of the registration contents and the disclosure range, consideration for financial support for clinical research by the government and the foundation of a public fund for that purpose, protecting the right of investigators in clinical research, presentation of what investigators should be and active guidance by MHLW and PMDA etc.

(3) Approval reviews
- Improvement of the qualification of reviewers, public announcement of instructions when imposing an approval condition, early submission of investigation results based on the approval condition carefully monitored and publication of the evaluation of the submitted information
- Ensuring transparency of the approval reviews by making open the discussion of the Council (PFSC) related to approval and incorporating more active disclosing procedures in the routine processes
- Consideration for shortening the period needed for the procedure in MHLW after completion of the review in PMDA, in order to speedily approve the drugs with high medical need as well as with the evidence
- Package inserts; Timely and periodic reflection of the latest knowledge on package insert and the advance confirmation procedure with the regulatory authority of its change, positioning as the official document and clarification of the administrative responsibility, and also scientific clarification of the range of efficacy (indications) based on evidence
- On the basis of the lessons learned that inappropriate off-label use caused drug-induced sufferings, drugs should be administered off-label only when the patient's benefit is really ensured with his/her consent and based on evidence.
- Drug companies, government and academic societies should play positive roles to obtain approval of necessary off-label use. In addition, economic support should be provided for clinical trials with high medical need.
- Revisit of the reevaluation system; setting a time limit in rebuttal by drug companies, and establishing the system where periodical review of the contents of package inserts is made based on the latest scientific knowledge

(4) Post-marketing risk management (safety measures)
- Stimulation of ADR reports etc. from medical institutions, setting up of the system utilizing the

ンに沿って「医薬品安性全監視の方法」を取り入れた「医薬品リスク管理」の実施。
- 電子レセプトデータベースなどのデータベースを活用して，副作用等の発現に関する医薬品使用者数や投薬情報を踏まえた安全対策(リスク管理)を講じることができ，その効果を評価できるような情報基盤を整備する。その際，個人情報保護を含めた情報の倫理的取り扱いに関するガイドラインを策定すべきである。
- 患者とのリスクコミュニケーション(リスクに関する情報提供)の円滑な実施：患者からの副作用報告制度の創設，患者向け情報資材の充実，苦情解決部門の設置，行政から提供される安全性情報の緊急性・重大性に応じた提供方法の見直し，予防原則に基づくグレー情報の伝達，医療機関の臨床現場への情報伝達が確実に実現できる体制の構築，患者への情報発信の強化，文書管理の徹底
- 一定の副作用の発現について個々の患者がその発現を早期に知ることができ，その結果として適切な治療を受けることができるような仕組み，診療明細の患者への発行の義務化，薬害の発生が確認された後の国民への情報伝達・公表の在り方，電子レセプトデータベースを活用した患者本人への通知方法及び起こりうる問題の検討
- 製薬企業による営利目的の不適切な情報提供や広告ならびに質の高いMR(医薬情報担当者)の育成に関する行政の指導監督
- GMP査察を実施する人材の確保，地方自治体が行うGMP査察の充実，GVPやGQP調査を実施する地方自治体の薬事監視員の資質向上及び人数確保に係わる国の配慮
- 個人輸入される未承認医薬品については，関連データのデータベース化と公表，副作用情報についての注意喚起と未承認医薬品の広告の監視・取締の強化，リスクが高い医薬品を個人輸入する医師の登録の要請，副作用情報の積極的な収集，その他の安全対策(リスク管理)の充実と強化
- インターネットを通じた未承認薬の個人輸入に関する規制の強化
- 患者数が極めて少ないという理由で企業による承認申請が順調に進まない未承認薬が国内に存在する。このような薬を適正に使用するため，「コンパッショネート・ユース」などの人道的な医薬品の使用手続きによる例外的使用システムを構築すべきである。ただし，かえって薬害を引き起こすことにならないよう慎重な検討と制度設計が必要である。

(5) 医療機関における安全対策(リスク管理)
- 医療機関は，健康被害の発生と薬害を防止するという観点からの積極的な取組により一定の役割を担うべきであり，そのための薬剤師の人員確保や育成を行うこと。
- 医療機関の安全管理責任者が主導する安全対策の体制強化，総合機構が提供している電子メールによる情報配信サービスへの登録の推進，チーム医療の推進による安全対策と薬剤師の積極的な安全対策への関与
- 医療機関内での適応外使用については，定期的点検，後日の点検が可能な仕組みの検討，適応外使用を含めたEBMガイドラインの作成と普及
- 医薬品情報を取り扱う部門が医薬品の安全性に関する情報を収集・評価し，その結果を医療現場に伝達する体制の構築，ならびに，実施状況を検証するための仕組みの構築

adverse reaction information from patients, reinforcement of international cooperation such as dispatch of the residence staff to the foreign regulatory authorities, standardization of adverse reaction report data internationally, and the system in the future where various safety information in medical settings are collected and evaluated in an integrated manner, and they lead to risk management activities

- Establishment of the system in which teams for each therapeutic category consisted of experts of medicine, pharmaceutical sciences, pharmacoepidemiology and biostatistics analyze and evaluate safety information collected for approval review and during post-marketing consistently, implementation of data mining activities, and promotion of investigation and research on pharmacogenomics
- Publication of safety information prior to the confirmation of its causality based on precautionary principle, and establishment of the risk management system for that purpose
- Introduction of "Risk minimization plan implementation system" (tentative name) which requires the company to submit a plan describing important points of post-marketing risk management and its management procedure from the stage of approval review, and to implement it appropriately after approval. In addition, implementation of "Drug risk management" incorporating "Pharmacovigilance Methods" in line with ICH-E2E guideline
- Development of information infrastructure with which safety measures (risk management) based on the number of drug users and/or medication information regarding the occurrence of ADRs etc. can be taken as well as their effect can be evaluated should be promoted, making use of databases such as the electronic receipt database. On that occasion, the guidelines about the ethical handling of information including personal information protection should be developed.
- Smooth implementation of risk communication with patients; Foundation of adverse reaction reporting system from patients, enrichment of information materials for patients, setting up the complaint solution section, review of the communication method of safety information offered by the administration corresponding its emergency and magnitude, communication of gray information based on precautionary principle, establishment of the system in which intensive communication up to clinical settings in medical institutions is secured, reinforcement of the information communication to patients, complete document management
- How individual patients can know the occurrence of certain adverse drug reactions in an early stage by which appropriate treatment can be taken, making it mandatory to issue medical fee bill to patients, how the information on drug-induced sufferings should be disclosed and communicated to the nation after its confirmation, consideration on a notifying method to the patient him/herself by utilizing an electronic receipt database and on possible problems involved
- Government's guidance and supervision regarding the inappropriate information communication and advertisement for profit by drug companies, and fostering highly qualified MRs (medical representatives)
- Securing human resources who conduct GMP inspection, reinforcement of GMP inspection by local governments, consideration by the government regarding the improvement of quality of and ensuring

(6) 健康被害救済制度
- 健康被害救済制度の周知徹底と，抗がん剤やその他の医薬品など救済対象となる医薬品の範囲の見直しの検討

(7) 専門的な知見を有効に活用するための方策
- 医薬品の安全性と有効に関するエビデンスの構築とその普及に向けて，学会の主導性の発揮

(8) 製薬企業に求められる基本精神
- 新薬開発の競争が激化しつつある現状を鑑みると，製薬企業に対してはこれまで以上にモラルが求められることが指摘された。
- 製薬企業も予防原則を基本とすることが強く求められており，製造販売後安全対策（リスク管理）をなお一層改善する必要があり。また，人員の適切な配置などの安全対策を強化し，後日の検証を可能にするための記録作成と保管を行う必要がある。
- 製薬企業における薬害教育，企業倫理委員会の設置など業界内部の自主的な倫理管理の充実と強化，利益相反関係の適切な管理

sufficient number of the pharmaceutical inspectors in local governments conducting GVP and/or GQP examinations
- Unapproved drugs privately imported; Database compilation and the publication of the data, raising awareness on the adverse reaction information and reinforcement of monitor and control of the advertisement on them, registration required of the doctors who import high-risk drug products privately, active collection of adverse reaction information, enrichment and reinforcement of other safety measures (risk management)
- Strengthening of the regulation regarding private import of unapproved drugs through Internet
- There are such domestically unapproved drugs whose approval applications do not proceed well by companies because of their extremely little number of patients. To make these drugs used properly, a system for exceptional use should be established by way of humanitarian drug use procedure such as "compassionate use". But careful examination and the system design are necessary not to rather cause drug-induced sufferings.

(5) Safety measures (risk management) in medical institutions
- Medical institutions should take certain roles by active efforts from the viewpoint of prevention of health damage occurrence and drug-induced sufferings, ensuring the number of and fostering pharmacists for that purpose.
- The system reinforcement of safety measures led by safety management supervisors in medical institutions, promoting registration to e-mail alert service by PMDA, safety measures by the promotion of team medicine, proactive participation of pharmacists in them
- Off-label use in medical institutions; Periodic check, studying mechanism under which future inspection is possible, preparation of EBM guidelines including off-label use and promotion of their wide use
- Establishment of the system in which the section dealing with drug information collects and evaluates information about drug safety and communicates the results to medical settings, as well as establishment of the mechanism to verify the situation of its implementation.

(6) Adverse health effects relief system
- Publicizing the adverse health effects relief system as best one can, and considering the review of the range of drugs eligible for relief, such as anti-cancer drugs and others

(7) Measures to utilize professional knowledge effectively
- Demonstration of the leadership from academic societies sought in development of the evidence on drug safety and efficacy and its wide use

(8) Basic spirit required for drug companies
- It was pointed out that morals were demanded for drug companies more than before just because it is the time when new drug development becomes increasingly competitive.
- Drug companies are also strongly demanded to be based on precautionary principle and

V．医薬品行政を担う組織の今後の在り方（概要）

(1) 医薬品行政組織について
- 「中間報告書」では，承認審査，安全対策，副作用被害救済等の業務を一括して厚生労働省医薬食品局が行い，審議会（薬事・衛生食品審議会：PFSC）が大臣へ答申を提出するという計画（A案）と，これらの業務すべてを総合機構が行うという計画（B案）に基づいて，課題が議論された。「第一次提言」には，引き続き医薬品行政のあるべき組織形態を検討していく旨が記載された。
- 2009年度に，厚生労働省医薬食品局（食品安全部を除く）の職員及び総合機構の職員に対してアンケート調査を実施した。
- 医薬品行政を一元化するのか，もしするのであればその役割を担うべきは国か独立行政法人かという点については結論が出なかった。しかし，アンケート調査の結果を踏まえ，以下の事項が指摘された：
    - 最終的には国が責任を負いその権限を適切に行使できる体制，安全対策に重点を置きながら承認審査と安全対策との一貫性を確保，全過程における透明性や職員の広い視野と専門性を確保，国民の声や医療現場の情報が適時適切に伝わる仕組み，医療政策との連携，企業に過度に依存しない収入源，必要な人員の確保と適切な人事システム，組織の在り方を絶えず検証・評価できる体制，厚生労働省と総合機構の役割分担を明確化

(2) 第三者監視・評価組織の創設
- 医薬品行政について，新たに，監視・評価機能を果たすことができる第三者的な組織を設置することが必要である（以下の具体的な在り方が指摘された）。
    - （目的）薬害の未然防止を目的として，医薬品行政機関とその活動に対して監視及び評価を実施する。
    - （特性）「独立性」「専門性」「機動性」
    - （権限）医薬品行政機関に対して，全般的な視点からの，また，個々の医薬品の安全性についての監視・評価を実施し，薬害防止のために適切な措置を講じるよう提言を行う。
    - （具体的権限）
        - ・厚生労働省及び総合機構から医薬品の安全性に関する情報を定期的に受領する。
        - ・行政機関に対して資料の提出を要求し，行政機関を通して製薬企業や医療機関から情報を収集する。

there's a need for more improvement in post-marketing safety measures (risk management), reinforcement of safety activities such as appropriate placement of the staff and documenting and archiving to enable future inspection.
- Education about drug-induced sufferings in drug companies, enrichment and reinforcement of the industry's voluntary ethics management such as establishing corporate ethics committee, and appropriate management of conflict of interest relations

V. Desirable structure of organization bearing the drug administration in the future (summary)

(1) On drug administrative organization
- In the "interim report", the issue was discussed based on the plan that Pharmaceutical and Food Safety Bureau of MHLW performs services such as approval reviews, safety measures, and adverse reaction relief etc. collectively and the Council (PFSC) submits the report to the minister (plan A) and the plan that PMDA performs all these services (plan B). In "the primary proposal" it was described that the desirable organizational form of drug administration would be examined continuously.
- Questionnaire survey of the staffs of Pharmaceutical and Food Safety Bureau of MHLW (except Department of Food Safety) and of PMDA was conducted in FY2009.
- We didn't reach a conclusion on whether to unify the drug administration and if so, such function should be vested in the government or in an independent administrative agency. However, based on the questionnaire results, the followings were pointed out :
  - System in which the government eventually takes responsibility and is able to exercise its authorities adequately, securing consistency between the approval reviews and safety measures while putting an emphasis on the latter, ensuring transparency in all processes, and broad perspective and specialties among staff, system in which voices of the people and information from medical practices come through timely and appropriately, cooperation with the medical policy, income sources which are not dependent on companies excessively, ensuring necessary number of staffs and appropriate personnel system, system under which how the organization should be can be verified and evaluated consistently, and clarifying the role sharing between MHLW and PMDA.

(2) The foundation of a third-party monitoring and evaluating body
- On drug administration, it is necessary to newly establish a third-party body which can fulfill its monitor and evaluation functions (the following specific points were made)
  - (Purpose) For the purpose of prevention of drug-induced sufferings, to monitor and evaluate drug administrative organizations and their activities
  - (Characteristics) "Independence", "Specialty" and "Mobility"
  - (Authority) To monitor and evaluate the drug administrative organizations in general and on the safety of individual drug products, and to make proposal to take appropriate measures for the prevention of drug-induced sufferings

・収集した情報に基づいて医薬品の安全性を評価する。
・収集した情報の監視・評価の結果に基づいて行政機関に対して提言を行う(行政機関は，自らが講じた対策の結果を報告する)。
◆ (位置付け)独立した委員から成る合議体(委員会または審議会)
・厚生労働省から独立した組織が望ましい。
・早急な実現が困難であれば，当面，厚生労働省内に当該第三者組織を設置することを提案する。この場合，その組織の独立性を確保するため，既存の審議会とは異なる仕組みが必要である。
◆ (構成委員)薬害被害者，市民(医薬品ユーザー)，医師，薬剤師，医薬品評価専門家，法律家，医薬品製造の専門家，マネージメントシステム専門家，倫理に関する専門家，薬剤疫学専門家など，委員長を含めて10名あるいはそれ以下
・上記のほか，例えば創設から3年ごとに，よりよい第三者組織の在り方を絶え間なく検討することが必要である。

- ◆ (Specific authorities)
    - · To periodically receive information on safety of drug products from MHLW and PMDA
    - · To demand presentation of materials from the administrative organizations, to collect information from drug companies or medical institutions through the administrative organizations
    - · To evaluate safety of the drug product based on the collected information
    - · To make proposals to the administrative organizations based on results of monitoring and evaluation (The organizations report the results of their actions.)
- ◆ (Positioning) Collegial body which consists of independent members (a committee or a council)
    - · The organization independent of MHLW is desirable.
    - · If its immediate realization is difficult, setting up the organization in MHLW for the time being is proposed. In this case, a different structure from the existing councils is necessary to secure its independence.
- ◆ (Member) Ten or less people including a chairperson, such as a person who has suffered from a drug-induced injury, citizen (drug user), doctor, pharmacist, drug evaluation expert, lawyer, drug manufacturing professional, management system expert, expert on ethics, and pharmacoepidemiologist etc.
    - · Other than the above, it is necessary to study how the third-party body should be better continuously, for example, in every three years after its foundation.

緊急安全性情報(イエローレター)と発出の実績

　緊急安全性情報は，米国のドクターレターに相当すると日本では考えられています。文字通り差し迫った状況から，各医療機関に伝達されます。緊急安全性情報は発出の理由，根拠となる事例紹介，安全対策(添付文書改訂など)から構成されます。その発出は厚生労働省が製薬企業に指示を行い，企業が作成してMRによる伝達が基本です。このほか，厚生労働省からのFAX一斉同送，厚生労働省のホームページへの掲載，マスコミを通じた国民への周知が同時に行われます。マスコミへの資料は，主として厚生労働省が作成します。

　このほか安全性速報(ブルーレター)と呼ばれるものは，緊急安全性情報に準じ，一般的な使用上の注意改訂(通常一か月以内の伝達)により迅速な安全対策措置をとる場合に発出されます。

　緊急安全性情報の1997年から2012年まで16年間の実績は以下の通りです。
◇2012年　9月11日：ランマーク®皮下注120mgによる重篤な低カルシウム血漿について
◇2004年　3月　5日：インスリン自己注射用注入器オプチペン®プロ1の使用に伴う過量投与の防止について
◇2003年　9月10日：経口腸管洗浄剤による腸管穿孔及び腸閉塞について
◇2003年　3月17日：ガチフロ錠100mg投与による低血糖及び高血糖について
◇2002年10月28日：精神病剤セロクエル25mg錠，同100mg(フマル酸クエチアピン)投与中の血糖値上昇による糖尿病性ケトアシドーシス及び糖尿病性昏睡について
◇2002年10月15日：イレッサ®錠250(ゲフィチニブ)による急性肺障害，間質性肺炎について
◇2002年　4月16日：抗精神病薬ジプレキサ®錠(オランザピン)投与中の血糖値上昇による糖尿病性ケトアシドーシス及び糖尿病性昏睡について
◇2000年11月15日：インフルエンザ脳炎・脳症患者に対するジクロフェナクナトリウム製剤の使用について
◇2000年10月　5日：塩酸ピオグリタゾン投与中の急激な水分貯留による心不全について
◇2000年　2月23日：尿酸排泄薬ベンズブロマロンによる劇症肝炎について
◇1999年　6月30日：塩酸チクロピジン製剤による血栓性血小板減少性紫斑病について
◇1998年12月18日：ウインセフ点滴用投与中の痙攣，意識障害について
◇1998年　8月　7日：オダイン錠(フルタミド)による重篤な肝障害について
◇1997年12月　1日：ノスカール(トログリタゾン)による重篤な肝障害について
◇1997年　8月14日：抗菌処理カテーテルを使用した際に発生したアナフィラキシーショックについて

Previously Issued Urgent Safety Information (Yellow Letter)

An Urgent Safety Information (Yellow Letter) in Japan may correspond to a "Dear Doctor" Letter in the US. As it literally means, it is communicated to individual medical institutions in case of significantly urgent circumstances. The Urgent Safety Information consists of the reason(s) for its issuance, introduction of the cases raising the necessity of issuance, and safety measures adopted (e.g. revision of package inserts). The basic flow is as follows: the Ministry of Health, Labour and Welfare (MHLW) orders a particular pharmaceutical company to issue an Urgent Safety Information; the company prepares the Yellow Letter; and its Medical Representatives (MRs) distribute it to medical institutions. At the same time, the MHLW sends by facsimile the information to healthcare professionals all at once, puts it on its web site, and makes it public thoroughly through the mass media. The document distributed to the mass media is primarily prepared by the MHLW.

In addition, a Rapid Safety Communication (Blue Letter) is issued, in accordance with the procedures for the Urgent Safety Information, by a particular pharmaceutical company given the order by the MHLW when prompt safety measures are taken due to a general revision of precautions for use (usually communicated within one month after the revision).

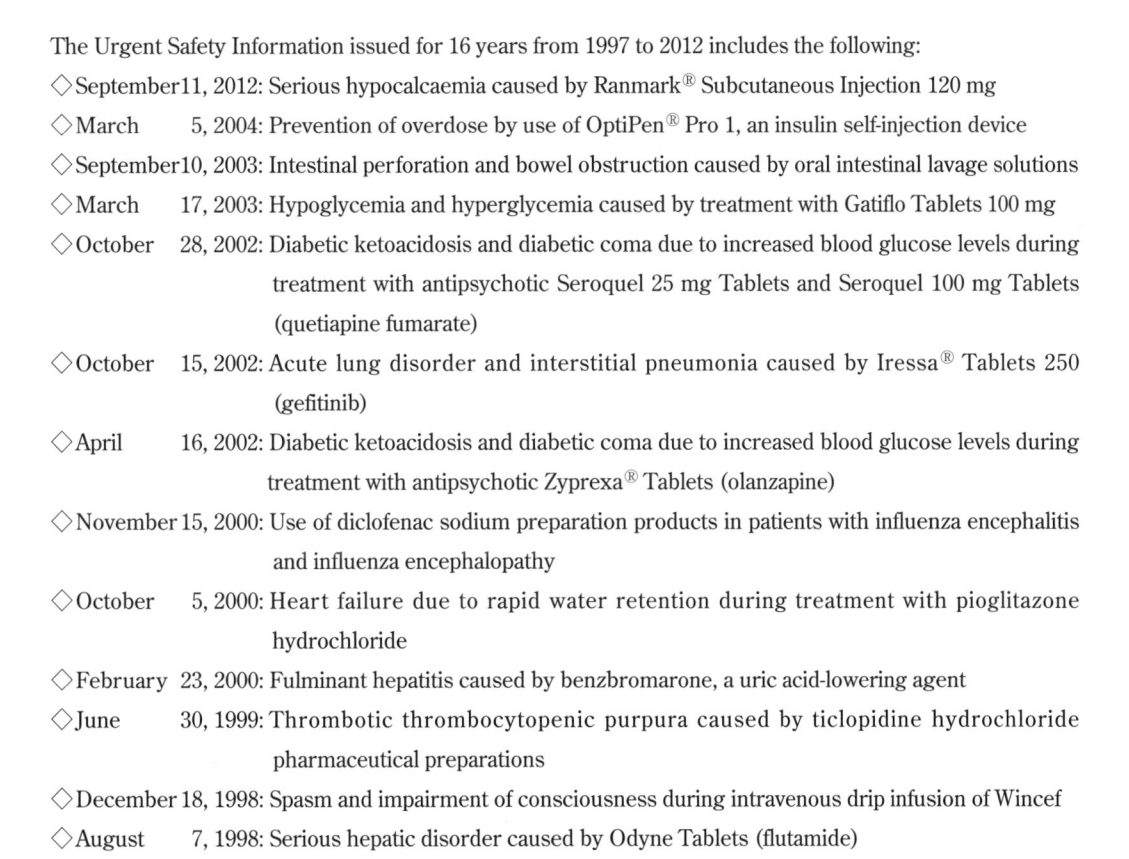

The Urgent Safety Information issued for 16 years from 1997 to 2012 includes the following:
- ◇ September 11, 2012: Serious hypocalcaemia caused by Ranmark® Subcutaneous Injection 120 mg
- ◇ March 5, 2004: Prevention of overdose by use of OptiPen® Pro 1, an insulin self-injection device
- ◇ September 10, 2003: Intestinal perforation and bowel obstruction caused by oral intestinal lavage solutions
- ◇ March 17, 2003: Hypoglycemia and hyperglycemia caused by treatment with Gatiflo Tablets 100 mg
- ◇ October 28, 2002: Diabetic ketoacidosis and diabetic coma due to increased blood glucose levels during treatment with antipsychotic Seroquel 25 mg Tablets and Seroquel 100 mg Tablets (quetiapine fumarate)
- ◇ October 15, 2002: Acute lung disorder and interstitial pneumonia caused by Iressa® Tablets 250 (gefitinib)
- ◇ April 16, 2002: Diabetic ketoacidosis and diabetic coma due to increased blood glucose levels during treatment with antipsychotic Zyprexa® Tablets (olanzapine)
- ◇ November 15, 2000: Use of diclofenac sodium preparation products in patients with influenza encephalitis and influenza encephalopathy
- ◇ October 5, 2000: Heart failure due to rapid water retention during treatment with pioglitazone hydrochloride
- ◇ February 23, 2000: Fulminant hepatitis caused by benzbromarone, a uric acid-lowering agent
- ◇ June 30, 1999: Thrombotic thrombocytopenic purpura caused by ticlopidine hydrochloride pharmaceutical preparations
- ◇ December 18, 1998: Spasm and impairment of consciousness during intravenous drip infusion of Wincef
- ◇ August 7, 1998: Serious hepatic disorder caused by Odyne Tablets (flutamide)

◇1997年　8月　6日：CPI社製ペースメーカーにおけるペーシング不全について
◇1997年　7月28日：塩酸イリノテカンと骨髄機能抑制について

◇December 1, 1997: Serious hepatic disorder caused by Noscar (troglitazone)
◇August 14, 1997: Anaphylactic shock which occurred during use of antibacterial-treated catheters
◇August 6, 1997: Pacing failure of pacemakers manufactured by CPI Company
◇July 28, 1997: Irinotecan hydrochloride and bone marrow suppression

薬食安発0411第1号
薬食審査発0411第2号
平成24年4月11日

各都道府県衛生主管部(局)長 殿

厚生労働省医薬食品局安全対策課長

厚生労働省医薬食品局審査管理課長

医薬品リスク管理計画指針について

　医薬品の安全性の確保を図るためには，開発の段階から製造販売後に至るまで常に医薬品のリスクを適正に管理する方策を検討することが重要です。特に新医薬品の製造販売後早期における医薬品安全性監視活動については，その計画の立案を支援することを意図して，「医薬品安全性監視の計画について」（平成17年9月16日付け薬食審査発0916001号・薬食安発0916001号厚生労働省医薬食品局審査管理課長・安全対策課長連名通知)を示してきました。このたび，医薬品安全性監視計画に加えて，医薬品のリスクの低減を図るためのリスク最小化計画を含めた，「医薬品リスク管理計画」を策定するための指針を別添のとおり取りまとめましたので，御了知のうえ貴管下関係業者に対し周知方御配慮願います。
　この指針は，新医薬品及びバイオ後続品については平成25年4月1日以降製造販売承認申請する品目から適用し，後発医薬品については適用時期を別途通知します。

＊本通知の英訳は医薬品医療機器総合機構によるものである。

PFSB/SD Notification No. 0411-1
PFSB/ELD Notification No. 0411-2
April 11, 2012

To: Directors of Prefectural Health Departments (Bureaus)

From: Directors of Safety Division
Pharmaceutical and Food Safety Bureau,
Ministry of Health, Labour and Welfare

Director of Evaluation and Licensing Division,
Pharmaceutical and Food Safety Bureau,
Ministry of Health, Labour and Welfare

Risk Management Plan Guidance

To ensure the safety of drugs, it is important to consider the ways to manage the risk of drugs on a consistent basis from the development phase to the post-marketing phase. In particular, to support the planning of pharmacovigilance activities in the early post-marketing phase of new drugs, MHLW previously issued a notification entitled "Pharmacovigilance Planning" (PFSB/ELD Notification No. 0916001 and PFSB/SD Notification No. 0916001 dated September 16, 2005, issued jointly by the Director of Evaluation and Licensing Division and the Director of Safety Division, Pharmaceutical and Food Safety Bureau, Ministry of Health, Labour and Welfare). In addition to this Pharmacovigilance Plan, MHLW have now formulated Guidance for development of a "Risk Management Plan," including a risk minimization plan to reduce the risk of drugs, as shown in the Annex. Please inform marketing authorization holders (MAHs) under your jurisdiction of this Notification.

This Guidance shall be applicable to new drugs and follow-on biologics for which approval applications are submitted on or after April 1, 2013. As for generic drugs, the timing of application of this Guideline shall be informed separately.

（別添）

医薬品リスク管理計画指針
目次

1. 緒言
    1.1 目的
    1.2 適用範囲

2. 医薬品リスク管理計画
    2.1 医薬品リスク管理計画の策定
    2.2 医薬品リスク管理計画の策定における留意事項
    2.3 医薬品リスク管理計画の節目となる予定の時期の設定
    2.4 医薬品リスク管理計画の見直し

3. 安全性検討事項
    3.1 安全性検討事項の特定
        3.1.1 重要な特定されたリスク
        3.1.2 重要な潜在的リスク
        3.1.3 重要な不足情報
    3.2 安全性検討事項の見直し

4. 医薬品安全性監視計画
    4.1 通常の医薬品安全性監視活動
    4.2 追加の医薬品安全性監視活動
    4.3 追加の医薬品安全性監視活動の実施計画

5. 有効性に関する調査・試験の計画

6. リスク最小化計画
    6.1 通常のリスク最小化活動
    6.2 追加のリスク最小化活動
        6.2.1 医療関係者への追加の情報提供
        6.2.2 患者への情報提供
        6.2.3 医薬品の使用条件の設定
        6.2.4 その他の活動
    6.3 追加のリスク最小化活動の実施計画

7. 医薬品リスク管理計画の評価及び総合機構への報告

(Annex)

Risk Management Plan Guidance
Table of Contents

1. **Introduction**
   1.1 Objective
   1.2 Scope

2. **Risk Management Plan**
   2.1 Development of Risk Management Plan
   2.2 Points to Consider in Development of Risk Management Plan
   2.3 Setting of Milestones in Risk Management Plan
   2.4 Review of Risk Management Plan

3. **Safety Specification**
   3.1 Identification of Safety Specification
      3.1.1 Important Identified Risks
      3.1.2 Important Potential Risks
      3.1.3 Important Missing Information
   3.2 Review of Safety Specification

4. **Pharmacovigilance Plan**
   4.1 Routine Pharmacovigilance Practices
   4.2 Additional Pharmacovigilance Activities
   4.3 Implementation Plan for Additional Pharmacovigilance Activities

5. **Plan for Survey/Study on Efficacy**

6. **Risk Minimization Plan**
   6.1 Routine Risk Minimization Practices
   6.2 Additional Risk Minimization Activities
      6.2.1 Provision of Additional Information to Healthcare Professionals
      6.2.2 Provision of Information to Patients
      6.2.3 Establishment of Conditions of the Use of the Drug
      6.2.4 Other Activities
   6.3 Implementation Plan for Additional Risk Minimization Activities

7. **Evaluation of Risk Management Plan and Report to PMDA**

1. 緒言

1.1 目的

　医薬品の承認時や製造販売後に，重要な特定されたリスク，重要な潜在的リスク及び重要な不足情報を安全性検討事項(Safety Specification)として集約し，それを踏まえて医薬品安全性監視活動の計画(医薬品安全性監視計画)を立てることについては，「医薬品安全性監視の計画について」(平成17年9月16日付け薬食審査発0916001号・薬食安発0916001号厚生労働省医薬食品局審査管理課長・安全対策課長連名通知。以下「ICH E2Eガイドライン」という。)により示され，対応が行われてきた。

　この指針は，ICH E2Eガイドラインに示されている安全性検討事項及びそれを踏まえた医薬品安全性監視計画に加えて，医薬品のリスクの低減を図るためのリスク最小化計画を含めた，医薬品リスク管理計画(RMP：Risk Management Plan)を策定するための基本的な考え方を示すものである。

　この指針を活用することにより，医薬品の開発段階，承認審査時から製造販売後の全ての期間において，ベネフィットとリスクを評価し，これに基づいて必要な安全対策を実施することで，製造販売後の安全性の確保を図ることを目的とする。

　なお，この指針の適用に当たっては，新医薬品，バイオ後続品又は後発医薬品など，それぞれの医薬品の特性を考慮した対応が必要である。

1.2 適用範囲

　この指針は，後発医薬品及びバイオ後続品を含む医療用医薬品を対象とする。

　具体的には，以下に示す時点に，この指針を基に医薬品リスク管理計画の策定を検討する。

○ 新医薬品(薬事法(昭和35年法律第145号。以下「法」という。)第14条の4第1項第1号に規定する新医薬品をいう。以下同じ。)の承認申請を行おうとする時点

○ バイオ後続品の承認申請を行おうとする時点

○ 追加の医薬品安全性監視活動又は追加のリスク最小化活動(以下「追加の措置」という。)が実施されている先発医薬品に対する後発医薬品の承認申請を行おうとする時点

○ 医薬品の製造販売後において，新たな安全性の懸念が判明した時点

2. 医薬品リスク管理計画

2.1 医薬品リスク管理計画の策定

　医薬品の製造販売業者又は製造販売承認申請者は，常に医薬品の適正使用を図り，ベネフィット・リスクバランスを適正に維持するため，医薬品について3.に示すとおり安全性検討事項を特定し，これを踏まえて，4.に示す医薬品安全性監視計画及び6.に示すリスク最小化計画を策定し，また，必要に応じて5.に示す有効性に関する製造販売後の調査・試験の計画を策定し，これらの計画の全体を取りまとめた医薬品リスク管理計画書を作成する。

1. Introduction

1.1 Objective

According to "Pharmacovigilance Planning" (PFSB/ELD Notification No. 0916001 and PFSB/SD Notification No. 0916001 dated September 16, 2005, issued jointly by the Director of Evaluation and Licensing Division and the Director of Safety Division, Pharmaceutical and Food Safety Bureau, Ministry of Health, Labour and Welfare; hereinafter referred to as the "ICH E2E Guideline"), it is required that the plan for pharmacovigilance activities (Pharmacovigilance Plan) is developed at the time of approval review and in the post-marketing phase based on the Safety Specification into which "important identified risks," "important potential risks," and "important missing information" are consolidated , and this instruction has been followed.

This Guidance is intended to present a basic concept for development of the Risk Management Plan that contains a risk minimization plan to reduce the risk of drugs in addition to the Safety Specification and Pharmacovigilance Plan described in the ICH E2E Guideline.

The objective of this Guidance is to ensure safety of drugs in the post-marketing phase by implementing the guidance and taking necessary safety measures based on a benefit-risk evaluation performed throughout the development, approval review and post-marketing phases.

This Guidance should be used taking into consideration the characteristics of individual drugs and their categories, such as new drugs, follow-on biologics, and generic drugs.

1.2 Scope

This Guidance is applicable to ethical use drugs, including generic drugs and follow-on biologics.

Based on this Guidance, development of the risk management plan should be considered at the following milestones:

○ At the time of submission of approval application for new drugs (the term "new drugs" means new drugs as defined in Article 14-4, paragraph (1), item (i) of the Pharmaceutical Affairs Law [Law No. 145, 1960; hereinafter referred to as "the Law"]; the same shall apply hereinafter);

○ At the time of submission of approval application for follow-on biologics;

○ At the time of submission of approval application for generic drug versions of the original drugs for which additional pharmacovigilance activities or additional risk minimization activities (hereinafter referred to as "additional actions") are being performed;

○ At the time when new concerns regarding safety have been identified in the post-marketing phase.

2. Risk Management Plan

2.1 Development of Risk Management Plan

In order to always promote proper use of drugs and maintain an appropriate risk-benefit balance, MAHs and applicants for marketing authorization should identify the Safety Specification of drugs as described in section 3, and develop a Pharmacovigilance Plan as described in section 4 and a Risk Minimization Plan as described in section 6 based on the identified Safety Specification. When necessary, they should also develop a plan for post-marketing survey/study on efficacy as described in section 5. The MAHs and applicants for marketing authorization should then prepare a Risk Management Plan by consolidating these plans.

2.2 医薬品リスク管理計画の策定における留意事項

医薬品リスク管理計画の策定に当たっては，安全性検討事項に応じて，通常の医薬品安全性監視活動及び通常のリスク最小化活動に加えて，追加の措置の必要性を検討し，それらを実施するか否かについて，その理由や手法とともに医薬品リスク管理計画書に明確に記載する。なお，医薬品リスク管理計画については，承認審査の過程においてその妥当性が検討されることになるので，その検討の内容を反映するため，審査報告書の記載内容との整合性を図って整備すること。

追加の措置の必要性を検討するに当たって考慮する点として，例えば以下の事項が挙げられる。
- 推定使用患者数
- 投与状況
- 特定されているリスク集団
- 対象疾患の重篤性，合併症の重篤性及び背景発現率
- 副作用がベネフィット・リスクバランス又は保健衛生の状況に対して及ぼす影響の大きさ
- 重篤な副作用の重症度，頻度，可逆性及び予防可能性
- リスク最小化活動の実施により期待される効果
- 海外での開発又は製造販売の状況
- 海外との安全性プロファイルの相違
- 海外で実施されている調査・試験の状況及び結果
- 海外で執られた安全対策

安全性検討事項を踏まえた医薬品リスク管理計画の検討の結果として，追加の措置が必要でないと判断される医薬品においても，通常の医薬品安全性監視活動として，法第77条の4の2に基づく副作用及び感染症情報の収集，報告等，並びに通常のリスク最小化活動としての添付文書等による情報提供の適切な実施が義務付けられていることに留意する。

2.3 医薬品リスク管理計画の節目となる予定の時期の設定

医薬品リスク管理計画の策定に当たっては，各医薬品安全性監視活動及びリスク最小化活動について，その結果の評価又は独立行政法人医薬品医療機器総合機構（以下「総合機構」という。）への報告を行う節目となる予定の時期を，各活動ごとに設定し，医薬品リスク管理計画書に記載する。

節目となる予定の時期は，各医薬品安全性監視活動及びリスク最小化活動ごとに設定するが，例えば，一つの活動で複数の安全性検討事項に関する検討を行う場合には，それぞれの安全性検討事項に関する目標を適切な時期に達成することができるように，各安全性検討事項に対応した節目となる評価又は報告の予定の時期を設定し，活動全体の進捗状況及び個別の安全性検討事項に係る進捗状況を管理できるようにする。

節目となる予定の時期を設定するに当たって考慮する点として，例えば以下の事項が挙げられる。
- 有害事象について事前に設定しておいた頻度を十分な信頼性をもって検出できるようになる時期はいつか
- 有害事象の発現に影響を及ぼすリスク因子を十分な正確さで評価できるようになる時期は

2.2 Points to Consider in Development of Risk Management Plan

When developing a Risk Management Plan, the necessity of additional actions should be considered at the same time as routine pharmacovigilance practices and routine risk minimization practices depending on the Safety Specification. A clear description should be provided in the Risk Management Plan about whether these actions are taken or not, together with the reasons and the methods. Because the validity of the Risk Management Plan is to be assessed during the approval review processes, in order to reflect the contents of the assessment of the Risk Management Plan, this Plan should be prepared so that consistency with the contents of the review reports be included.

As points of consideration for the necessity of additional actions, the followings are examples of them:

○ Estimated number of patients to be treated with the drug;
○ Situation or status of the drug administration;
○ Identified risk population;
○ Seriousness of target disease, seriousness of complications, and background incidence rate;
○ Degree of influence of adverse drug reactions (ADRs) on the benefit-risk balance or public health conditions;
○ Severity, frequency, reversibility, and possibility of prevention of serious ADRs;
○ Effects expected from implementing risk minimization activities;
○ Development or marketing situations in overseas;
○ Differences in safety profiles between Japan and overseas;
○ Situations and results of survey/study performed in overseas;
○ Safety measures taken in overseas.

It should be noted that, even for drugs for which additional actions have been judged unnecessary as a result of considering the Risk Management Plan based on the Safety Specification, routine pharmacovigilance practices (including collection and reporting of information regarding ADRs and infections) as stipulated in Article 77-4, paragraph (2) of the Law and routine risk minimization practices (including provision of information through package inserts etc.) must be appropriately performed.

2.3 Setting of Milestones in Risk Management Plan

When developing a Risk Management Plan, the milestones for evaluating the results or for reporting to the Pharmaceuticals and Medical Devices Agency (hereinafter referred to the "PMDA") should be established by individual pharmacovigilance activities and risk minimization activities and be described on an activity-by-activity basis in the Risk Management Plan.

Although the milestones are to be established individually for pharmacovigilance activities and risk minimization activities, this plan of milestones should be the one that makes the management of the progress of overall activities and the progress of individual items of the Safety Specifications possible; for example, when examining more than one item of the Safety Specification in one activity, a milestone for evaluation or reporting of each item of Safety Specification should be established so that the target of each item of the Safety Specification be achieved at an appropriate time point.

The points to consider when setting the milestones include, for example, the following:

いつか
- 実施中又は実施を計画している医薬品安全性監視活動の結果を利用することができるようになる時期はいつか
- リスク最小化活動の対象としている安全性検討事項に関する臨床上及び保健衛生上の重要性が評価できるようになる時期はいつか(安全性検討事項が非常に重要なものである場合には，リスク最小化活動の効果について，その評価をより早期に，かつ，頻繁に行うこと)

2.4 医薬品リスク管理計画の見直し

医薬品リスク管理計画を一度策定した後にも，製造販売後の状況に応じて適切に見直しを行い，医薬品のベネフィット・リスクバランスを適正に維持するよう，その内容を改訂する必要がある。

医薬品リスク管理計画に含まれるそれぞれの医薬品安全性監視活動及びリスク最小化活動の実施状況に応じて見直しを行うことが必要であり，例えば以下の時点が挙げられる。
- 製造販売後に新たな安全性の懸念が判明した場合など，安全性検討事項の内容に変更があった時
- 医薬品リスク管理計画で設定している節目となる時期
- 規制に基づく又は総合機構から指示されている定期的な報告の時期
- 新医薬品の再審査申請を行う時

3. 安全性検討事項

3.1 安全性検討事項の特定

それぞれの医薬品について，有効成分，剤型等の薬剤としての特徴，対象疾患，投与対象となる患者群等の特性を考慮し，安全性検討事項の特定を行う。

安全性検討事項の特定は，その医薬品における特定されたリスク，潜在的リスク及び不足情報のうち，ヒトにおいて発現した場合に重篤である，又は高頻度に発現する等の理由から，当該医薬品のベネフィット・リスクバランスに影響を及ぼしうる，又は保健衛生上の危害の発生若しくは拡大のおそれがあるような重要なものについて，重要な特定されたリスク，重要な潜在的リスク及び重要な不足情報として要約した安全性検討事項を特定することが求められる。

安全性検討事項の特定については，ICH E2Eガイドラインを参照すること。

3.1.1 重要な特定されたリスク

医薬品との関連性が十分な根拠に基づいて示されている有害な事象のうち重要なものをいう。特定されたリスクは，例えば以下のものが挙げられる。
- 非臨床試験において医薬品との関連性が十分に明らかにされており，臨床データにおいても確認されている副作用及び感染症(以下「副作用等」という。)

○ When will it become possible to detect the predetermined frequency of adverse events (AEs) with sufficient reliability?
○ When will it become possible to evaluate risk factors that affect the onset of AEs with sufficient accuracy?
○ When will it become possible to use the results of pharmacovigilance activities that are being performed or planned?
○ When will it become possible to evaluate the clinical and health importance of the items of the Safety Specification that are the targets of risk minimization activities? (If the Safety Specification is critical, evaluation of the effects of risk minimization activities should be conducted earlier and more frequently.)

2.4 Review of Risk Management Plan

Even after the Risk Management Plan has been developed, it should be reviewed depending on the post-marketing situations, and the contents of the Risk Management Plan should be revised to maintain an appropriate benefit-risk balance of the drug.

The review of the Risk Management Plan should be performed depending on the situations of individual pharmacovigilance activities and risk minimizing activities included in the Plan. The examples of the timing of this review are listed below:

○ When the content of the Safety Specification needs to be changed; for example, at the time when new safety concerns have been identified after marketing;
○ At a predetermined milestone in the Risk Management Plan;
○ At the time of periodic reporting based on regulations or as directed by the PMDA;
○ At the time of re-examination application for new drugs.

3. Safety Specification

3.1 Identification of Safety Specification

The Safety Specification should be identified for individual drugs in view of the properties of the drug such as the active ingredient and dosage form, characteristics of target diseases and the patient population to be administered the drug, etc..

It is required to identify the Safety Specification which comprises the summary of important identified risks, important potential risks, and important missing information among identified risks, potential risks, and missing information of the pertinent drug. These important identified risks, important potential risks, and important missing information are critical in that they may affect the benefit-risk balance of the drug or may cause or increase public health hazards on grounds such as they may become serious if they occur in humans or frequently occur.

For identification of Safety Specification, reference should be made to the ICH E2E Guideline.

3.1.1 Important Identified Risks

These are defined as important AEs among AEs for which the association with the drug is shown based

- 適切に設計された臨床試験や疫学研究において，比較対照群との相違から医薬品との因果関係が示された副作用等
- 製造販売後に多くの自発報告があり，これらにより時間的関連性や生物学的妥当性から因果関係が示唆される副作用等

3.1.2 重要な潜在的リスク

医薬品との関連性が疑われる要因はあるが，臨床データ等からの確認が十分でない有害な事象のうち重要なものをいう。潜在的リスクは，例えば以下のものが挙げられる。
- 非臨床データから当該医薬品の安全性の懸念となり得る所見が示されているが，臨床データ等では認められていない事象
- 臨床試験や疫学研究において，比較対照群との相違から医薬品との因果関係が疑われるが，十分に因果関係が示されていない有害事象
- 製造販売後に自発報告から生じたシグナルとして検出された当該医薬品との因果関係が明らかでない有害事象
- 当該医薬品では認められていないが，同種同効薬で認められている副作用等
- 当該医薬品の薬理作用等の性質から発現が予測されるが，臨床データ等では確認されていない事象

3.1.3 重要な不足情報

医薬品リスク管理計画を策定した時点では十分な情報が得られておらず，製造販売後の当該医薬品の安全性を予測する上で不足している情報のうち重要なものをいう。不足情報は，例えば以下のものが挙げられる。
- 治験の対象から除外されていた患者集団であるが，実地医療で高頻度での使用が想定される等の理由により，当該患者集団での安全性の検討に必要となる情報

3.2 安全性検討事項の見直し

医薬品の製造販売業者は，ICH E2Eガイドラインに基づき，常に当該医薬品の安全性検討事項について見直しを行う必要がある。製造販売後の医薬品安全性監視活動等の結果として，新たな安全性の懸念が判明したときは，速やかに安全性検討事項の内容を見直す。安全性検討事項を変更するときは，医薬品リスク管理計画の見直しを行い，医薬品リスク管理計画書をはじめとした関連する文書を整備する等，必要な措置を行う。

on sufficient evidence. Identified risks include, for example, the following:
- ○ ADRs or infections (hereinafter referred to as "ADRs etc.") for which the association with the drug has been well established in non-clinical studies and confirmed by clinical data;
- ○ ADRs etc. for which causal relationship with the drug has been shown by the difference with the control group in well-designed clinical studies or epidemiological studies;
- ○ ADRs for which causal relationship is suggested by temporal relationship or biological rationality derived from many spontaneous reports in the post-marketing phase.

3.1.2 Important Potential Risks

These are defined as important AEs among AEs for which the association with the drug has been suspected due to some factors but not been sufficiently confirmed by clinical data etc.. Potential risks include, for example, the following:
- ○ Events that have not been observed by clinical data etc. although there are findings of safety concerns of the drug in non-clinical data;
- ○ AEs for which causal relationship with the drug is not sufficiently shown, although causal relationship is suspected by the difference with the control group in clinical trials or epidemiological studies;
- ○ AEs that have been detected as a signal from spontaneous reports in the post-marketing phase and have unclear causal relationship with the drug;
- ○ ADRs etc. which have not been observed in the drug but have been observed in drugs of the same class with the same indications;
- ○ Events that have not been confirmed in the clinical data etc., although the onset of the AEs are predicted from the properties of the pharmacological effects of the drug.

3.1.3 Important Missing Information

These are defined as critical information in cases where sufficient information has not been obtained at the time of development of the Risk Management Plan, and thus information is missing for prediction of safety in the post-marketing phase of the drug. Missing information includes, for example, the following:
- ○ Information that is necessary for evaluating the safety in a certain patient population excluded from the clinical study, because, for example, high frequency use of the drug in this patient population is anticipated in real-world practice setting.

3.2 Review of Safety Specification

MAHs should always review the Safety Specification of the drug according to the ICH E2E Guideline. When new safety concerns have emerged as a result of post-marketing pharmacovigilance activities etc., the contents of the Safety Specification should be immediately reviewed. When the Safety Specification is amended, necessary measures (e.g. review of the Risk Management Plan and revision of related documents including the Risk Management Plan) should be taken.

4. 医薬品安全性監視計画

　医薬品安全性監視計画については，ICH E2Eガイドラインを参照し，以下を踏まえてその内容を検討する。

4.1　通常の医薬品安全性監視活動

　製造販売業者において実施している通常の医薬品安全性監視活動及びその実施体制について要約する。

4.2　追加の医薬品安全性監視活動

　安全性検討事項を踏まえて，追加の医薬品安全性監視活動の必要性，その理由，手法等について検討の上，その実施体制とともに要約する。医薬品安全性監視活動の手法については，医療情報データベースを活用した薬剤疫学的手法も含め，ICH E2Eガイドラインの別添「医薬品安全性監視の方法」を参照するほか，以下のことも考慮する。

- ○ 新医薬品においては，販売開始直後において，稀で重篤な副作用が見出されることがあるので，医療機関に対し確実な情報提供，注意喚起等を行い，適正使用に関する理解を促すとともに，重篤な副作用等の情報を迅速に収集し，必要な安全対策を実施し，副作用等の被害を最小限にすることが重要である。このため，必要に応じ，追加の医薬品安全性監視活動として，市販直後調査の実施が求められる。市販直後調査については，「医薬品，医薬部外品，化粧品及び医療機器の製造販売後安全管理の基準に関する省令」（平成16年厚生労働省令第135号），「医療用医薬品の市販直後調査の実施方法等について」（平成18年3月24日付け薬食安発第0324001号厚生労働省医薬食品局安全対策課長通知）等の関連する法令，通知等を参照すること。
- ○ 医薬品の製造販売後に，法第77条の4の2に基づく副作用等報告による情報が集積され，新たに重篤又は致死的な副作用等が判明するなど，新たな安全性の懸念が判明し，安全性検討事項が変更されることがある。この場合において，追加のリスク最小化活動が実施された場合には，そのリスク最小化活動の効果の評価のために追加の医薬品安全性監視活動の必要性も検討する。
- ○ 当該医薬品の適応となる患者集団において，原疾患やその合併症の自然経過といった背景の中で発現率の高い有害事象がある場合には，それが当該医薬品による副作用等との鑑別が困難なこともある。そのような場合にも，追加の医薬品安全性監視活動の必要性を検討する。

　なお，新たに特定された安全性検討事項に基づいて，追加の医薬品安全性監視活動を計画し，実施する場合には，事前に総合機構と相談を行うこと。

4.3　追加の医薬品安全性監視活動の実施計画

　追加の医薬品安全性監視活動を実施する場合においては，医薬品リスク管理計画書の作成又は改訂を行う。医薬品リスク管理計画書には，各医薬品安全性監視活動について，以下の事項等を含んだ概要を簡潔に記載する。また，各医薬品安全性監視活動の詳細について実施計画書を作成する。

- ○ 実施計画書の表題

4. Pharmacovigilance Plan

The content of the Pharmacovigilance Plan should be considered based on the following, using the ICH E2E Guideline as a reference.

4.1 Routine Pharmacovigilance Practices

MAHs should summarize their routine pharmacovigilance practices and their implementation system.

4.2 Additional Pharmacovigilance Activities

The necessity, the reasons, methods, etc. of additional pharmacovigilance activities should be considered based on the Safety Specification and summarized with the implementation system. For the methods of pharmacovigilance activities including pharmacoepidemiological methods utilizing a healthcare information database, reference should be made to the "Pharmacovigilance Methods" in the Annex of the ICH E2E Guideline. In addition, the following points should be considered:

- ○ Because rare and serious ADRs of new drugs may be observed early in the post-marketing phase, it is important that MAHs ensure to provide medical institutions with correct information and alerts about it, and remind them to promote understanding of proper use, collect information of serious ADRs etc. quickly, take necessary safety measures, and minimize health hazards from the ADRs etc. Therefore, if necessary, Early Post-marketing Phase Vigilance is required as additional pharmacovigilance activities. As for Early Post-marketing Phase Vigilance, reference should be made to relevant laws, regulations, and notifications, such as "Ministerial Ordinance on Good Vigilance Practice (GVP) for drugs, quasi-drugs, cosmetics, and medical devices" (Ordinance of the Ministry of Health, Labour and Welfare No. 135, 2004) and "Implementation Methods for Early Post-marketing Phase Vigilance for Prescription Drugs" (PFSB/SD Notification No. 0324001 of the Safety Division, Pharmaceutical and Food Safety Bureau, Ministry of Health, Labour and Welfare; dated March 24, 2006).
- ○ In the post-marketing phase, new safety concerns, such as serious or fatal ADR, may be identified by accumulated information from ADR reports pursuant to Article 77-4-2 of the Law, and thus the Safety Specification may need to be modified. If this happens and the MAHs have implemented additional risk minimization activities, they are also required to conduct additional pharmacovigilance activities to evaluate the effect of the risk minimization activities.
- ○ If the incidence rates of AEs in a patient population to be treated with the drug are high, and if the background incident rates of the AEs in this population are also considered high because of the natural course of the primary disease or complications, it may be difficult to determine whether or not the AEs are ADRs of the drug. When this type of situation occurs, the need for conducting additional pharmacovigilance should be considered.

If MAHs are to plan and conduct additional pharmacovigilance activities based on the newly identified Safety Specification issues, they should preliminarily consult with the PMDA.

4.3 Implementation Plan for Additional Pharmacovigilance Activities

When additional pharmacovigilance activities are implemented, a Risk Management Plan should be prepared or revised. A summary including the following items regarding the individual pharmacovigilance activities should be

○ 安全性検討事項
○ 当該医薬品安全性監視活動の実施計画(案)
○ 当該医薬品安全性監視活動の目的
○ 当該医薬品安全性監視活動の実施計画の根拠
○ 当該医薬品安全性監視活動の結果に基づいて実施される可能性のある追加の措置及びその開始の決定基準
○ 当該医薬品安全性監視活動の実施状況及び得られた結果の評価，又は総合機構への報告を行う節目となる予定の時期及びその根拠

複数の安全性検討事項に対し，一つの医薬品安全性監視活動で対応する場合にはその旨を記載する。

なお，製造販売後臨床試験を行う場合においては，安全性検討事項に関するモニタリングの詳細及び試験中止についての規定を記載する。また，必要に応じて，「医薬品の臨床試験の実施の基準に関する省令」(平成9年厚生省令第28号)第19条に規定する効果安全性評価委員会への情報提供及び当該試験の中間解析の実施時期を医薬品リスク管理計画書に記載する。

医薬品安全性監視活動として実施する調査・試験・研究において，有効性に関する情報収集を行う場合には，その旨を記載する。

5. 有効性に関する調査・試験の計画

医薬品の有効性に関する情報の収集を目的として調査，試験等を実施する場合には，当該調査等を実施する目的，その手法等について4.3を参考にして簡潔にその要約を記載する。なお，医薬品安全性監視計画の策定においても有効性に関する情報の収集を考慮すること。

6. リスク最小化計画

リスク最小化計画とは，医薬品の承認時までに得られた情報及び当該医薬品の製造販売後に医薬品安全性監視活動により収集された安全性等に関する情報並びにそれらの情報の評価に基づき，当該医薬品のリスクを最小に抑え，ベネフィット・リスクバランスを適切に維持するために実施する個々のリスク最小化活動の全般を束ねたものをいう。リスク最小化活動は，全ての医薬品において通常行われる活動と，当該医薬品の特性等を踏まえ，必要に応じて通常のリスク最小化活動に追加して行われる活動がある。

6.1 通常のリスク最小化活動

医薬品の用法，用量，効能，効果等の製造販売承認事項及び当該医薬品の使用上の注意を記載した法第52条に規定する添付文書を作成し，また，必要に応じて改訂し，その内容を医療関係者に対して情報提供することは，通常行われるべきリスク最小化活動であり，その実施体制と併せて通常のリスク最小化活動として要約する。

また，「「患者向医薬品ガイドの作成要領」について」(平成17年6月30日付け薬食発第

briefly described in the Risk Management Plan. In addition, a detailed implementation plan for individual pharmacovigilance activities should be prepared.
- ○ Title of the implementation plan;
- ○ Safety Specification;
- ○ Implementation plan for the pharmacovigilance activities of the drug (draft);
- ○ Objective of the pharmacovigilance activities of the drug;
- ○ Rationale for the implementation plan of the pharmacovigilance activities of the drug
- ○ Possible additional actions to be taken based on the results of the pharmacovigilance activities of the drug and the decision criteria for initiating them;
- ○ Milestones for evaluating the implementation status and the results of the pharmacovigilance activities of the drug or for reporting them to the PMDA, and the rationale for the milestones.

When more than one item of the Safety Specification is dealt with by a single pharmacovigilance activity, this should be described.

When post-marketing clinical trials are conducted, the details of monitoring regarding the Safety Specification and rules on discontinuation of the study should be described. When necessary, the milestones of providing information to the Efficacy and Safety Assessment Committee specified in Article 19 of the "Ministerial Ordinance on Good Clinical Practices" (Ordinance of the Ministry of Health and Welfare No. 28, 1997) and of interim analyses of the trial should be described in the Risk Management Plan.

When information regarding efficacy is collected through surveys, trials, or studies as part of pharmacovigilance activities, this should be described.

5. Plan for Survey/trials on Efficacy

When a survey/trial is conducted to collect efficacy information of the drug, a summary of the objective of and the methods for the survey/trial should be briefly described using section 4.3 as a reference. In addition, collection of efficacy information should be taken into consideration when developing the Pharmacovigilance Plan.

6. Risk Minimization Plan

The risk minimization plan refers to the consolidated individual risk minimization activities conducted to minimize the risk of the drug and to maintain a appropriate benefit-risk balance based on information obtained by the time of approval, information on safety and others collected through the post-marketing pharmacovigilance activities, and evaluation of the information. The risk minimization activities are classified into two categories; i.e., routine activities conducted for all drugs and additional activities conducted, if necessary, according to the characteristics of the product in addition to the routine risk minimization practices.

6.1 Routine Risk Minimization Practices

Routine risk minimization practices include preparing package inserts describing approved items such as "Dosage and Administration""Indications" and "Precautions" as specified in Article 52 of the Law, revising them as necessary, and providing information of the contents to healthcare professionals. The contents of these practices together with the implementation system should be summarized as the routine risk minimization practices.

In addition, the Drug Guide for Patients prepared based on the "Guideline for Developing the Drug Guide

06300001号厚生労働省医薬食品局長通知)及び「患者向医薬品ガイドの運用について」(平成18年2月28日付け薬食安発第0228001号・薬食監麻発第0228002号厚生労働省医薬食品局安全対策課長・監視指導・麻薬対策課長連名通知)に基づき作成される患者向医薬品ガイドは，通常のリスク最小化活動とする。

6.2 追加のリスク最小化活動

追加のリスク最小化活動としては，例えば，以下に示すような，通常行われる添付文書情報の提供に加えて，特に安全性検討事項について行われる医療関係者への情報提供，当該医薬品の投与対象となる患者への情報提供，当該医薬品の使用条件の設定等がある。個別の医薬品の特性等に応じて，これらのリスク最小化活動の実施の必要性及び組合せを検討し，追加のリスク最小化計画を策定する。

6.2.1 医療関係者への追加の情報提供

○ 市販直後調査による情報提供

市販直後調査は，当該医薬品の適正使用に関する理解を促すとともに，重篤な副作用等の情報を迅速に収集し，必要な安全対策を実施し，副作用等の被害を最小限にすることを目的として，医薬品の販売開始後の6か月間行われるもので，4.2に示したとおり追加の医薬品安全性監視活動であるとともに，医療機関に対し確実な情報提供，注意喚起等を行う，追加のリスク最小化活動でもある。

○ 適正使用のための資材の作成及び配布

安全性検討事項に関連し，医薬品の適正使用を医療関係者に対し周知するため，総合機構と協議のうえ，適正使用のための資材を作成し，配布する。

○ 製造販売後の医薬品安全性監視活動により得られた情報の迅速な公表

安全性検討事項に関し，医薬品の使用に際して特段の注意が必要な場合等においては，製造販売後の医薬品安全性監視活動により得られた副作用等の集積状況等を当該医薬品の製造販売業者等の特定の利用者のみ対象としたものではないホームページにおいて公表し，適切な頻度で更新を行う等により，医療関係者に対する周知を行う。この際には，関係学会等との連携を図ることや，総合機構の医薬品医療機器情報提供ホームページにも掲載を行うこと等も考慮する。

○ その他

安全性検討事項に関連する関係学会等の第三者の作成する適正使用を目的としたガイドライン等が存在する場合には，それらを活用して情報提供する。

6.2.2 患者への情報提供

○ 安全性検討事項に応じた資材の作成及び提供

安全性検討事項に関連し，総合機構と協議のうえ，医薬品の特性等に応じて，患者手帳等の個別の注意点等を記載した患者向け資材を作成し，提供する。

for Patients" (PFSB Notification No. 06300001 of the Director-General of Pharmaceutical and Food Safety Bureau, Ministry of Health, Labour, and Welfare; dated June 30, 2005) and the "Use of the Drug Guide for Patients" (Joint PFSB/SD Notification No. 0228001and PFSB/CND Notification No. 0228002 issued jointly by the Director of Safety Division and the Director of Compliance and Narcotics Division, Pharmaceutical and Food Safety Division, Ministry of Health, Labour and Welfare; dated February 28, 2006) should be regarded as part of the routine risk minimizing practices.

6.2 Additional Risk Minimization Activities

Additional risk minimization activities include, for example, provision of information, especially on the Safety Specification, to healthcare professionals, provision of information to the patients to be treated with the drug, and establishment of conditions for the use of the drug as described below, in addition to routine provision of package insert information. The MAHs should consider the necessity of implementation of these risk minimization activities or combinations of them depending on the characteristics etc. of individual drugs, and develop an additional risk minimization plan.

6.2.1 Provision of Additional Information to Healthcare Professionals

○ Provision of information based on Early Post-marketing Phase Vigilance

Early Post-marketing Phase Vigilance is conducted during the first six months from the time of initial marketing to promote understanding of the proper use of the drug and minimize the harm of ADRs etc. by collecting information on serious ADRs etc. and taking necessary safety measures. It is also part of the additional pharmacovigilance activities as described in section 4.2 as well as the additional risk minimization activities that ensure to provide information and alerts etc. to medical institutions.

○ Preparation and provision of materials for proper use

Regarding the Safety Specification, MAHs should consult with the PMDA and prepare materials for the proper use of the drug and provide them to healthcare professionals to ensure that they are well aware of the proper use.

○ Rapid release of information obtained by post-marketing pharmacovigilance activities

Regarding the Safety Specification, when particular caution should be exercised regarding the use of the drug, MAHs should release the accumulated information such as the ADRs etc. which was obtained through the post-marketing pharmacovigilance activities on the their websites which are not targeted to limited users, and update the information at an appropriate frequency to ensure that healthcare professionals are well aware of the information. The MAHs should also consider working together with academic associations etc. and also publishing the information on the PMDA website.

○ Others

If available, MAHs may use guidelines etc. on the proper use of the drugs, prepared by third parties, such as academic associations relevant to Safety Specification issues.

6.2.3 医薬品の使用条件の設定

医薬品の特性や対象疾患の性質等に鑑み，適正使用による安全性の確保を目的として，必要に応じて使用に当たっての条件を設定する。医薬品の製造販売業者は，当該使用条件を確保し得る医療機関に対して医薬品を納入する等，製造販売に当たって必要な措置を講ずる。これらの条件は，医薬品の添付文書の使用上の注意への記載，承認条件としての規定，安全管理手順等の一環としての規定等の形で設定される。例えば以下のものが挙げられる。

○ 専門的知識・経験のある医師による使用の確保

治療域が狭い医薬品，重篤な副作用等が懸念される医薬品等については，医薬品を処方する医師に対して，対象疾患の治療に関する高度な専門的知識及び経験を求める。また，これに加えて，投与に際して特別な注意を要する医薬品については，医薬品の使用方法等に関する講習会の受講等，知識及び経験を確保するための一定の要件を定めた上で，製造販売業者における医師の登録等を求める。

○ 医薬品の使用管理体制の確保

重篤な副作用等により致命的な経過をたどる可能性がある医薬品，投与後の患者の状態の厳格な管理が必要な医薬品等については，緊急時に十分な対応が可能な医療機関での使用，入院管理下での投与等の使用管理体制の確保を求める。特別な薬剤管理が必要な医薬品については，管理体制の確保や，医師，薬剤師等の登録を求める。

○ 投与対象患者の慎重な選定

医薬品の有効性，安全性を確保する上で，投与対象となる患者を特に慎重に選定する必要がある医薬品については，患者の状態，既往歴，治療歴，併用薬等の状況を勘案した条件を設定する。特に注意を要する場合には，患者の条件への適合性に係る事前確認の確保やモニタリングの実施，医薬品の製造販売業者における投与患者の登録等を求める。

○ 投与に際しての患者への説明と理解の実施

医薬品の投与に伴い致命的な副作用等の発現リスクが高く，その早期発見やその際の主治医への連絡体制の確保等を図る上で，患者側の理解が特に必要とされる医薬品等については，投与に先立ち，患者及びその家族に対して医薬品の有効性，安全性等に関する説明を十分に行い，同意を得た上で投与する旨の条件を設定する。また，特定の重篤なリスクを回避するために，患者側の理解を補助し，注意を徹底するために患者向けの資材や教育プログラム等の提供を行う。

○ 特定の検査等の実施

医薬品の投与対象患者の適切な選択や，医薬品の使用により発現が予測される特定の副作用等を防止するため，医薬品の投与前又は投与後に特定の検査等を実施する旨の条件を設定する。

6.2.2 Provision of Information to Patients

○ Preparation and provision of materials according to the Safety Specification

Regarding the Safety Specification, MAHs should consult with the PMDA and prepare and provide materials for patients describing specific precautions etc., such as a patient handbook, depending on the characteristics of the drug.

6.2.3 Establishment of Conditions of the Use of the drug

MAHs should establish conditions of the use of the drug, as necessary, to ensure proper and safe use of the drug according to the properties of the drug or the nature of the disease. The MAHs should take appropriate measures in marketing the drug, such as distributing their products only to medical institutions that can meet the conditions of the use of the drugs. These conditions are established in the forms such as the description of Precautions in the package inserts of the drug, regulations as conditions for approval, and regulations as part of safety control procedures. The conditions of the use of the drug include, for example, the following:

○ Securing of use by physicians with sufficient expertise and experience

If drugs with a narrow therapeutic range or possible serious ADRs are to be used, MAHs should require prescribing physicians to have sufficiently high expertise and experience on the treatment of the disease. As for drugs that require special precautions for use, MAHs should also set certain requirements to secure physicians' expertise and experience, such as participation in a training session regarding the use of the drug etc., and require the physicians to register to the MAHs' program before using the drug.

○ Securing the management system of the use of the drug

As for drugs which may lead to fatal course associated with serious ADRs or require strict management of the conditions of patients after administration, MAHs should require healthcare professionals to secure the management system of the use of the drug such as the use of the drug only in medical institutions where sufficient emergency treatment is available or under hospitalization. In addition, for drugs requiring special management, securing of a management system and registration of physicians, pharmacists, etc. should be required.

○ Careful selection of treatment patients

For drugs that need careful selection of treatment patients to ensure efficacy and safety, MAHs should establish conditions by taking into consideration the conditions of patients, medical history, treatment history, concomitant drugs, etc. In cases where special caution needs to be exercised, pre-confirmation of the eligibility of the patients, monitoring, registration of the treatment patients to the MAHs' program, etc. are required.

○ Informed consent prior to administration of the drug

Regarding drugs that have a high risk of onset of fatal ADRs and especially require the understanding of patients to facilitate early detection of those ADRs or to ensure communication systems with their physicians, conditions for administration of these drugs should be established in a way that sufficient explanation on the efficacy, safety, etc. of the drug are given to the patients and their families and consent from them are received

6.2.4 その他の活動
○ 表示，容器・包装等の工夫
　　ヒューマンエラー防止等の観点から，医薬品の表示，容器・包装等に特別の措置を講じる。

6.3 追加のリスク最小化活動の実施計画
　追加のリスク最小化活動を実施する場合においては，医薬品リスク管理計画書の作成又は改訂を行う。医薬品リスク管理計画書には，実施中及び実施を計画している各リスク最小化活動について，以下の事項等を含んだ概要を簡潔に記載する。
○ 安全性検討事項
○ 当該リスク最小化活動の目的
○ 当該リスク最小化活動の具体的内容
○ 当該リスク最小化活動を実施する根拠
○ 当該リスク最小化活動の結果に基づいて実施される可能性のある追加の措置及びその開始の決定基準
○ 当該リスク最小化活動の実施状況及び得られた結果の評価，又は総合機構への報告を行う節目となる予定の時期及びその根拠

7．医薬品リスク管理計画の評価及び総合機構への報告
　各医薬品安全性監視活動，有効性に関する調査・試験及びリスク最小化活動については，医薬品リスク管理計画に基づき，実施状況及び得られた結果についての評価を，その節目となる時期に適切に行う。評価の際には，医薬品リスク管理計画に基づいて実施された各活動から得られた情報を踏まえて，医薬品のベネフィット・リスクバランスに関する評価及び考察も行う。
　再審査期間中の新医薬品については，法第14条の4第6項の規定又は法第14条の5第2項前段の規定による報告に係る薬事法施行規則（昭和36年厚生省令第1号）第63条に規定する安全性定期報告の際に，その評価内容を要約して報告し，その他の医薬品にあっては，追加の措置の内容に応じ，報告時期を医薬品リスク管理計画に規定する。
　この報告の際には，医薬品リスク管理計画の見直しについて，その検討結果も報告することとし，計画の変更を行う場合には，必要に応じ，事前に総合機構と相談を行う。報告の内容については，総合機構において確認を行い，何らかの対策が必要と判断された場合には，製造販売業者に対する指示が行われる。

prior to administration. In addition, to avoid specific serious risks, materials and educational programs for patients should be provided to assist the understanding of patients and their families and to ensure awareness of risks.

○ Specific tests etc.

In order to select patients who are appropriate for the treatment or to prevent specific possible ADRs etc. with the use of the drug, MAHs should establish conditions that certain tests etc. be performed before or after the administration of the drug.

6.2.4 Other Activities

○ Devising failsafe labeling, containers, packaging, etc.

Specific measures concerning labeling, containers, packaging, etc. may be taken to prevent human errors etc. from happening.

6.3 Implementation Plan for Additional Risk Minimization Activities

When implementing additional risk minimization activities, the Risk Management Plan should be prepared or revised. A summary of individual risk minimization activities being implemented or planned to be implemented including the following should be briefly described in the Risk Management Plan:

- ○ Safety Specification;
- ○ Objective of the risk minimization activities;
- ○ Specific contents of the risk minimization activities;
- ○ Rationale for implementing the risk minimization activities;
- ○ Possible additional actions to be taken based on the results of the risk minimization activities of the drug and the decision criteria for initiating them;
- ○ Milestones for evaluating the implementation status and results of the risk minimization activities of the drug or for reporting them to the PMDA, and the rationale for the milestones.

7. Evaluation of the Risk Management Plan and Report to the PMDA

The implementation status and the results of individual pharmacovigilance activities, surveys/trials on efficacy, and risk minimization activities should be evaluated appropriately at their respective milestones according to the Risk Management Plan. At the same time, the benefit-risk balance of the drug should also be evaluated and considered based on the information obtained from individual activities conducted according to the Risk Management Plan. As for new drugs which are in the re-examination period, a summary of the contents of evaluation should be reported at the time of submitting periodic safety reports as specified in Article 63 of the Enforcement Regulations (Ordinance of the Ministry of Health and Welfare No.1, 1961) regarding reports stipulated in Article 14-4, paragraph (6) or in the first half of Article 14-5, paragraph (2) of the Law. As for other drugs, the timing of reporting should be described in the Risk Management Plan depending on the contents of the additional actions.

The review results of the Risk Management Plan should also be reported together with the above report. If there are changes in the plan, MAHs should preliminarily consult with the PMDA, as necessary. The PMDA

checks the contents of the report, and if it considers that some measures should be taken, the PMDA will give directions to MAHs.

薬食審査発0426 第2号
薬食安発0426 第1号
平成24年4月26日
(平成25年3月4日付け薬食審査発0304 第1号
・薬食安発0304 第1号通知により一部改正)

各都道府県衛生主管部(局)長 殿

厚生労働省医薬食品局審査管理課長

厚生労働省医薬食品局安全対策課長

医薬品リスク管理計画の策定について

　「医薬品リスク管理計画」については，平成24年4月11日付け薬食安発0411第1号・薬食審査発0411 第2号厚生労働省医薬食品局安全対策課長・審査管理課長連名通知により，その指針を示しましたが，具体的な計画書の様式，提出等の取扱いについて下記のとおり示しますので，御了知のうえ，貴管下関係業者に対し周知方御配慮願います。
　なお，後発医薬品の取扱いについては，別途通知します。

記

1. 医薬品リスク管理計画書の作成について

(1) 医薬品リスク管理計画書は，別紙様式により作成すること。
(2) 医薬品リスク管理計画書は，一つの有効成分であれば，効能・効果，用法・用量，剤型，投与経路等の異なる製剤について，一つの計画書を作成することでも差し支えないこと。
(3) 複数の製造販売業者が共同で医薬品安全性監視活動及びリスク最小化活動を実施する場合には，連名で医薬品リスク管理計画書を提出しても差し支えないこと。その際，記載事項が品目により異なる場合においても同一の欄に，品目ごとの違いがわかるように記載すること。

PFSB/ELD Notification No. 0426-2
PFSB/SD Notification No. 0426-1
April 26, 2012
(Partially revised by PFSB/ELD Notification No. 0304-1
and PFSB/SD Notification No. 0304-1, both dated March 4, 2013)

To: Directors of Prefectural Health Departments (Bureaus)

From: Director of Evaluation and Licensing Division,
Pharmaceutical and Food Safety Bureau,
Ministry of Health, Labour and Welfare

Director of Safety Division,
Pharmaceutical and Food Safety Bureau,
Ministry of Health, Labour and Welfare

Development of Risk Management Plan

The Ministry of Health, Labour and Welfare (MHLW) previously formulated the Guidance for development of a "Risk Management Plan" under PFSB/SD Notification No. 0411-1 and PFSB/ELD Notification No. 0411-2 dated April 11, 2012, issued jointly by the Director of Safety Division and the Director of Evaluation and Licensing Division, Pharmaceutical and Food Safety Bureau, Ministry of Health, Labour and Welfare. The MHLW have now specified the form of Risk Management Plan and how to handle it, including among others, submission of the Plans, as described in the Notice section below. Please inform marketing authorization holders (MAHs) under your jurisdiction of this Notification.
Handling of generic drugs shall be informed separately.

Notice

1. Preparation of a Risk Management Plan

(1) Prepare a Risk Management Plan using the specified Form as shown in the Attachment to this Notification.

(2) It is acceptable to prepare a single Risk Management Plan for formulations different in indications, dosage and administration, dosage forms, administration routes, and other relevant aspects, provided that the formulations contain a single active ingredient.

(3) When more than one marketing authorization holder (MAH) cooperates with one another in conducting pharmacovigilance activities and risk minimization activities, it is acceptable to submit a Risk Management Plan jointly developed by the MAHs concerned. In such a case, even when

2. 承認申請時の医薬品リスク管理計画書の案の提出について

(1) 新医療用医薬品の承認申請に当たっては,「新医薬品の製造販売の承認申請に際し承認申請書に添付すべき資料の作成要領について」(平成13年6月21日付け医薬審発第899号厚生労働省医薬局審査管理課長通知)の記の第三のⅠ.1.(11)及び別紙2の11に示す製造販売後調査等基本計画書の案を提出することとしているが,平成25年4月1日以降に承認申請を行う品目については,製造販売後調査等基本計画書の案に代えて,別紙様式により作成した医薬品リスク管理計画書の案を提出すること。

なお,本通知日以降,製造販売後調査等基本計画書の案に代えて,承認申請書に添付する資料として医薬品リスク管理計画書の案を提出しても差し支えないこと。

(2) バイオ後続品の承認申請に当たっては,「バイオ後続品の品質・安全性・有効性確保のための指針」(平成21年3月4日付け薬食審査発第0304007号厚生労働省医薬食品局審査管理課長通知)の別添の9.に基づき製造販売後調査とリスク管理計画の具体的な方法や計画を提出することとしているが,平成25年4月1日以降に承認申請を行う品目については,これに代えて,別紙様式により作成した医薬品リスク管理計画書の案を提出すること。

なお,本通知日以降,製造販売後調査とリスク管理計画の具体的な方法や計画に代えて,承認申請書に添付する資料として医薬品リスク管理計画書の案を提出しても差し支えないこと。

3. 医薬品リスク管理計画書及び製造販売後調査等実施計画書の提出について

(1) ① 上記2の(1)により,承認申請時に,医薬品リスク管理計画書の案を提出した品目にあっては,「新医療用医薬品の再審査に係る製造販売後調査等基本計画書等について」(平成17年10月27日付け薬食審査発第1027007号厚生労働省医薬食品局審査管理課長通知)の3.に基づく製造販売後調査等基本計画書に代えて,医薬品リスク管理計画書を,原則として販売開始予定時期の1か月前までに,参考資料とともに提出すること。

② 上記2の(2)により,承認申請時にリスク管理計画書の案を提出した品目にあっては,製造販売後調査とリスク管理計画の具体的な方法や計画に代えて,医薬品リスク管

entries for a required matter differ depending on the products concerned, indicate the differences in the column for the matter so that the product-specific differences are clearly identified.

2. Submission of Draft Risk Management Plan upon Submission of Approval Application

(1) At the time of submission of approval applications for new prescription drugs, it shall be required to submit a draft Basic Plan for Post-Marketing Surveillance specified in Part 3-I. 1. (11) of the Notice of a notification entitled "Guidelines for Preparation of Data Attached to Applications for Approval to Manufacture or Import New Drugs" (PMSB/ELD Notification No. 899 dated June 21, 2001, issued by the Director of Evaluation and Licensing Division, Pharmaceutical and Medical Safety Bureau (PMSB), Ministry of Health, Labour and Welfare) and indicated also in Item 11 of Attachment 2 to the above-stated notification. As for products for which approval applications are submitted on and after April 1, 2013, however, a draft Risk Management Plan using the specified Form as shown in the Attachment to this Notification shall be submitted in place of a draft Basic Plan for Post-Marketing Surveillance.

On the date of issuance of this Notification onwards, it is acceptable to include a draft Risk Management Plan, in place of a draft Basic Plan for Post-Marketing Surveillance, in the data required for approval applications.

(2) At the time of submission of approval applications for follow-on biologics, it shall be required to submit the specific methods and plans for post-marketing surveillance and risk management planning as described in Section 9 of Attachment to a notification entitled "Guidance for Securing Quality, Safety, and Efficacy of Follow-on Biologics"(PFSB/ELD Notification No. 0304007 dated March 4, 2009, issued by the Director of Evaluation and Licensing Division, Pharmaceutical and Food Safety Bureau, MHLW). As for products for which approval applications are submitted on and after April 1, 2013, however, a draft Risk Management Plan using the specified Form as shown in the Attachment to this Notification shall be submitted in place of the above-stated specific methods and plans.

On the date of issuance of this Notification onwards, it is acceptable to include a draft Risk Management Plan, in place of the specific methods and plans for post-marketing surveillance and risk management planning, in the data required for approval applications.

3. Submission of Risk Management Plan and Implementation Plan for Post-Marketing Surveillance

(1) i) As for products for which draft Risk Management Plans are submitted at the time of submission of approval applications under (1) of the above Section 2, a Risk Management Plan shall be submitted in place of a Basic Plan for Post-Marketing Surveillance under Section 3 of a notification entitled "Basic Plan, etc. for Post-Marketing Surveillance concerning Reexamination of New Prescription Drugs" (PFSB/ELD Notification No. 1027007 dated October 27, 2005, issued by the Director of Evaluation and Licensing Division, Pharmaceutical and Food Safety Bureau, Ministry of Health, Labour and Welfare), as a rule at least one month prior to the

理計画書を，原則として販売開始予定時期の1か月前までに，参考資料とともに提出すること．
(2) 追加の医薬品安全性監視活動についての個別の製造販売後調査等実施計画書は，別添に掲げる事項を記載し，原則として調査又は試験の開始予定時期の1か月前までに提出すること．
(3) 提出方法は，独立行政法人医薬品医療機器総合機構（以下「総合機構」という）審査業務部業務第一課に直接持参又は郵送すること．
(4) 提出部数は，正本1部及び副本2部とすること．

4. 製造販売後に新たな安全性の懸念が判明した場合の医薬品リスク管理計画書の提出について

製造販売後に新たな安全性の懸念が判明し，医薬品リスク管理計画を作成・変更する場合の医薬品リスク管理計画書の提出時期や内容については，総合機構に相談すること．

5. その他

(1) 上記4の場合を含め，医薬品リスク管理計画の変更に当たっては，軽微な変更を除き，最新の医薬品リスク管理計画書を総合機構に提出すること．提出に当たっては，変更部分に下線を引くとともに，参考として直近の提出内容を併記すること．
(2) 医薬品リスク管理計画の実施に基づく定期的な報告の様式については，追って通知する．

scheduled date of initial marketing of the product concerned, together with reference data.

    ii) As for products for which draft Risk Management Plans are submitted at the time of submission of approval applications under (2) of the above Section 2, a Risk Management Plan, shall be submitted in place of the specific methods and plans for post-marketing surveillance and risk management planning, as a rule at least one month prior to the scheduled date of initial marketing of the product concerned, together with reference data.

(2) Individual Implementation Plans for Post-Marketing Surveillances regarding additional pharmacovigilance activities shall include the matters listed in the Attachment to this Notification and shall be submitted as a rule at least one month prior to the scheduled initiation of the surveillance or study concerned.

(3) The documents to be submitted shall be personally delivered or sent by mail to the Administration Division 1, Office of Review Administration, Pharmaceuticals and Medical Devices Agency (PMDA).

(4) One original copy and two duplicate copies of the document shall be submitted.

4. Submission of Risk Management Plan upon Receipt of New Safety Concerns Identified in the Post-Marketing Phase

When new concerns regarding safety have been identified in the post-marketing phase, requiring development of a Risk Management Plan or any change to the existing Risk Management Plan, the MAH concerned shall consult with the PMDA regarding the timing of submission of and the contents of a new or revised Risk Management Plan.

5. Others

(1) When any change is made to the existing Risk Management Plan, including those made under the above Section 4, the latest Risk Management Plan shall be submitted to the PMDA. This shall not apply to minor changes, though. In the latest version to be submitted, the changes made shall be underlined and for the purpose of reference, accompanied with the previous statements included in the Plan that has been submitted most recently.

(2) The form for periodic reporting on the basis of implementation of Risk Management Plans shall be informed later.

(別紙様式)

医薬品リスク管理計画書

平成　年　月　日

独立行政法人医薬品医療機器総合機構理事長 殿

　　　　　　　　　住所：(法人にあっては主たる事務所の所在地)
　　　　　　　　　氏名：(法人にあっては名称及び代表者の氏名)印

標記について次のとおり提出します。

品目の概要			
承認年月日		薬効分類	
再審査期間		承認番号	
国際誕生日			
販売名			
有効成分			
含量及び剤型			
用法及び用量			
効能又は効果			
承認条件			
備考			

ATTACHMENT

(Form)

Risk Management Plan

Date: _____ (Month) _____ (Day), _____ (Year)

To: Chief Executive of Pharmaceuticals and Medical Devices Agency

    Address: (For a corporation, indicate the location of its main office.)
    Name: (For a corporation, indicate its name and the name of its representative.) Seal

We hereby submit this Risk Management Plan as specified below.

Outline of Product				
Date of approval		Therapeutic class		
Period of reexamination		Approval No.		
International Birth Date				
Brand name				
Active ingredient				
Content and dosage form				
Dosage and administration				
Indication(s)				
Conditions for approval				
Remarks				

変更の履歴
前回提出日
変更内容の概要：
変更理由：

History of Changes
Date of the last submission
Summary of the change(s):
Reason(s) for the change(s):

1. 医薬品リスク管理計画の概要

1.1 安全性検討事項

重要な特定されたリスク
(重要な特定されたリスクの名称)
重要な特定されたリスクとした理由：
医薬品安全性監視活動の内容及びその選択理由：
リスク最小化活動の内容及びその選択理由：
(重要な特定されたリスクの名称)
重要な特定されたリスクとした理由：
医薬品安全性監視活動の内容及びその選択理由：
リスク最小化活動の内容及びその選択理由：
(重要な特定されたリスクの名称)
重要な特定されたリスクとした理由：
医薬品安全性監視活動の内容及びその選択理由：
リスク最小化活動の内容及びその選択理由：

1. Overview of Risk Management Plan

1.1 Safety Specification

Important Identified Risks
(Name of important identified risk)
Reason(s) why this is considered an important identified risk:
Contents of pharmacovigilance activities and reason(s) for selection of these activities:
Contents of risk minimization activities and reason(s) for selection of these activities:
(Name of important identified risk)
Reason(s) why this is considered an important identified risk:
Contents of pharmacovigilance activities and reason(s) for selection of these activities:
Contents of risk minimization activities and reason(s) for selection of these activities:
(Name of important identified risk)
Reason(s) why this is considered an important identified risk:
Contents of pharmacovigilance activities and reason(s) for selection of these activities:
Contents of risk minimization activities and reason(s) for selection of these activities:

重要な潜在的リスク		
(重要な潜在的リスクの名称)		
	重要な潜在的リスクとした理由：	
	医薬品安全性監視活動の内容及びその選択理由：	
	リスク最小化活動の内容及びその選択理由：	
(重要な潜在的リスクの名称)		
	重要な潜在的リスクとした理由：	
	医薬品安全性監視活動の内容及びその選択理由：	
	リスク最小化活動の内容及びその選択理由：	
(重要な潜在的リスクの名称)		
	重要な潜在的リスクとした理由：	
	医薬品安全性監視活動の内容及びその選択理由：	
	リスク最小化活動の内容及びその選択理由：	

Important Potential Risks
(Name of important potential risk)
Reason(s) why this is considered an important potential risk:
Contents of pharmacovigilance activities and reason(s) for selection of these activities:
Contents of risk minimization activities and reason(s) for selection of these activities:
(Name of important potential risk)
Reason(s) why this is considered an important potential risk:
Contents of pharmacovigilance activities and reason(s) for selection of these activities:
Contents of risk minimization activities and reason(s) for selection of these activities:
(Name of important potential risk)
Reason(s) why this is considered an important potential risk:
Contents of pharmacovigilance activities and reason(s) for selection of these activities:
Contents of risk minimization activities and reason(s) for selection of these activities:

重要な不足情報
(重要な不足情報の名称)
重要な不足情報とした理由：
医薬品安全性監視活動の内容及びその選択理由：
リスク最小化活動の内容及びその選択理由：
(重要な不足情報の名称)
重要な不足情報とした理由：
医薬品安全性監視活動の内容及びその選択理由：
リスク最小化活動の内容及びその選択理由：
(重要な不足情報の名称)
重要な不足情報とした理由：
医薬品安全性監視活動の内容及びその選択理由：
リスク最小化活動の内容及びその選択理由：

Important Missing Information
(Name of important missing information)
Reason(s) why this is considered important missing information:
Contents of pharmacovigilance activities and reason(s) for selection of these activities:
Contents of risk minimization activities and reason(s) for selection of these activities:
(Name of important missing information)
Reason(s) why this is considered important missing information:
Contents of pharmacovigilance activities and reason(s) for selection of these activities:
Contents of risk minimization activities and reason(s) for selection of these activities:
(Name of important missing information)
Reason(s) why this is considered important missing information:
Contents of pharmacovigilance activities and reason(s) for selection of these activities:
Contents of risk minimization activities and reason(s) for selection of these activities:

1.2 有効性に関する検討事項

(有効性に関する検討事項の名称)	
	有効性に関する検討事項とした理由：
	有効性に関する調査・試験の名称：
	調査・試験の目的，内容及び手法の概要並びに選択理由：

1.2 Efficacy-Related Issue

(Name of efficacy-related issue)	
	Reason(s) why this is an efficacy-related issue:
	Name of survey/trial on efficacy:
	Objective(s), contents, and outlined methods of the survey/trial as well as reasons for selection:

2. 医薬品安全性監視計画の概要

通常の医薬品安全性監視活動	
通常の医薬品安全性監視活動の概要：	
追加の医薬品安全性監視活動	
(医薬品安全性監視活動の名称)	
(医薬品安全性監視活動の名称)	
(医薬品安全性監視活動の名称)	

2. Overview of Pharmacovigilance Plan

Routine Pharmacovigilance Activities
Summary of routine pharmacovigilance activities:
Additional Pharmacovigilance Activities
(Name of pharmacovigilance activity)
(Name of pharmacovigilance activity)
(Name of pharmacovigilance activity)

3. 有効性に関する調査・試験の計画の概要

(有効性に関する調査・試験の名称)	

(有効性に関する調査・試験の名称)	

(有効性に関する調査・試験の名称)	

3. Overview of Plan for Survey/Trial on Efficacy

(Name of survey/trial on efficacy)

(Name of survey/trial on efficacy)

(Name of survey/trial on efficacy)

4. リスク最小化計画の概要

通常のリスク最小化活動
通常のリスク最小化活動の概要：

追加のリスク最小化活動
（リスク最小化活動の名称）
（リスク最小化活動の名称）
（リスク最小化活動の名称）

4. Overview of Risk Minimization Plan

Routine Risk Minimization Activities
Summary of routine pharmacovigilance activities:

Additional Risk Minimization Activities	
(Name of risk minimization activity)	
(Name of risk minimization activity)	
(Name of risk minimization activity)	

5. 医薬品安全性監視計画，有効性に関する調査・試験の計画及びリスク最小化計画の一覧

5.1 医薬品安全性監視計画の一覧

通常の医薬品安全性監視活動				
追加の医薬品安全性監視活動				
追加の医薬品安全性監視活動の名称	節目となる症例数／目標症例数	節目となる予定の時期	実施状況	報告書の作成予定日

5.2 有効性に関する調査・試験の計画の一覧

有効性に関する調査・試験の名称	節目となる症例数／目標症例数	節目となる予定の時期	実施状況	報告書の作成予定日

chapter 4 • REFERENCE DATA

5. At-a-Glance Tables for Pharmacovigilance Plan, Plan for Survey/Trial on Efficacy, and Risk Minimization Plan

5.1 At-a-Glance Table for Pharmacovigilance Plan

Routine Pharmacovigilance Activities				
Additional Pharmacovigilance Activities				
Name of additional pharmacovigilance activity	Milestone for No. of patients/target No. of patients	Milestone	Status of implementation	Scheduled date of development of report

5.2 At-a-Glance Table for Plan for Survey/Trial on Efficacy

Name of survey/trial on efficacy	Milestone for No. of patients/target No. of patients	Milestone	Status of implementation	Scheduled date of development of report

205

5.3 リスク最小化計画の一覧

通常のリスク最小化活動		
追加のリスク最小化活動		
追加のリスク最小化活動の名称	節目となる予定の時期	実施状況

5.3 At-a-Glance Table for Risk Minimization Plan

Routine Risk Minimization Activities		
Additional Risk Minimization Activities		
Name of additional minimization activity	Milestone	Status of implementation

6. 医薬品リスク管理計画のための組織体制

6.1 責任者

責任者	所属	氏名
安全管理責任者		
製造販売後調査等管理責任者		

6.2 安全管理業務のための組織体制

6.3 製造販売後調査等業務のための組織体制

7. 参考資料

6. Organizational System for Risk Management Plan

6.1 Individuals with Relevant Responsibilities

Responsible persons	Affiliation	Name
Safety management supervisor		
Supervisor of post-marketing surveys, etc.		

6.2 Organizational System for Fulfilling Safety Management Duties

6.3 Organizational System for Fulfilling Duties Involved in Post-Marketing Surveys, etc.

7. Reference Data

記載要領

1. 全般的事項について

- 用紙の大きさは日本工業規格A4とすること。
- 記載欄に記載事項の全てを記載できない場合には，その欄に「別紙○のとおり」と記載し，別紙を添付しても差し支えないこと。
- 計画書の各項目について，該当する事項がない場合には，その旨を記載することで差し支えないこと。
- 本計画書の案を承認申請の資料として提出する場合には，その時点での実施計画書及び資材の案の概要を併せて提出することが望ましいこと。
- 承認申請の時点以外で本計画書の案を提出する場合には，追加の医薬品安全性監視活動及び追加のリスク最小化活動に関する実施計画書及び資材の案を作成し，併せて提出すること。

2. 「品目の概要」について

- 本計画書の案を承認申請の資料として提出する場合には，「承認年月日」，「承認番号」，「承認条件」等の未定の項目については空欄とし，「薬効分類」，「用法及び用量」，「効能又は効果」等の項目については製造販売承認申請書に記載したものを「（予定）」として記載すること。
- 「備考」には，以下の事項を記載すること。
  ・再審査期間中，再審査期間終了，後発医薬品等の別
  ・担当者の氏名，所属，連絡先の電話番号等
  ・共同開発品目がある場合には，品目名及び会社名。ただし，本計画書を連名で提出する場合には，共同開発品目についての記載は不要であること。

3. 「医薬品リスク管理計画の概要」について

- 「安全性検討事項」について，重要な特定されたリスク，重要な潜在的リスク及び重要な不足情報がそれぞれ複数ある場合には，必要な数だけ欄を増やして記載すること。
- 「重要な特定されたリスクとした理由」，「重要な潜在的リスクとした理由」及び「重要な不足情報とした理由」について，非臨床データからの情報，臨床データからの情報，製造販売後の状況を踏まえ，適宜，関連する資料，文献等を添付して引用するなど，簡潔な記載に努めること。なお，承認申請の資料として本計画書の案を提出する場合には，コモン・

Instructions for Completing Risk Management Plan Form

1. General Matters

- The size of the paper shall be Japanese Industrial Standard A4.
- When all information to be indicated cannot be written within the prescribed column, it is acceptable to state "Refer to Attachment __" in that column and attach a separate sheet of paper containing all relevant information, to the Form.
- When there is no applicable information to be stated for a prescribed matter in the Plan, it is acceptable to indicate that fact in the column of the matter concerned.
- When a draft Risk Management Plan is to be submitted as the data required for approval application, it is desirable to submit, together with the draft Risk Management Plan, overviews of a draft implementation plan and a draft for materials, both available at the time of the above-stated submission.
- When a draft Risk Management Plan is to be submitted at the time other than that of submission of approval application, it is required to prepare implementation plans for both additional pharmacovigilance activities and additional risk minimization activities as well as a draft for materials, and submit these documents together with the draft Risk Management Plan.

2. Section "Outline of Product"

- When a draft Risk Management Plan is to be submitted as the data required for approval application, leave the columns for undetermined matters, e.g. "Date of approval", "Approval No.", and "Conditions for approval", blank. For matters such as "Therapeutic class", "Dosage and administration", and "Indication(s)", indicate the information stated in the approval application, and add "(Expected)" to the indicated information.
- State the following information in the column "Remarks":
  - Whether the product is being subject to a reexamination or has completed the reexamination period, or is a generic drug, and any other relevant information
  - The name, affiliation, telephone number for contact, and any other relevant information of the individual responsible for the product
  - When there exists any product under joint development of the product concerned, indicate the name of the jointly developed product and the name(s) of the company(ies) participating in the joint development. When the Risk Management Plan is to be submitted in the joint names, however, it is unnecessary to state the jointly developed product.

3. Section "Overview of Risk Management Plan"

- In the subsection "Safety Specification", increase the number of individual columns for important identified risks, important potential risks, and important missing information so that all such risks and information to be indicated will be included in the Form.
- In the columns "Reason(s) why this is considered an important identified risk", "Reason(s) why this is considered an important potential risk", and "Reason(s) why this is considered important missing information", take into account information from non-clinical data and clinical data as well as post-

テクニカル・ドキュメントの関連する項目との整合性を十分に考慮すること。
- ○「有効性に関する検討事項」が複数ある場合には，必要な数だけ欄を増やして記載すること。なお，該当する項目がない場合には記載は不要であること。
- ○ 医薬品安全性監視活動，有効性に関する調査・試験の実施又はリスク最小化活動が，承認条件，薬事・食品衛生審議会における指示事項等に基づく場合は，その旨を記載すること。

4.「医薬品安全性監視計画の概要」について

- ○ 追加の医薬品安全性監視活動について，それに係る安全性検討事項，目的，根拠等について記載すること。なお，追加の医薬品安全性監視活動が複数ある場合には，それぞれ必要な数だけ欄を増やして記載すること。
- ○ 追加の医薬品安全性監視活動がある場合には，その実施計画書を製造販売後調査等実施計画書として提出すること。

5.「有効性に関する調査・試験の計画の概要」について

- ○ 有効性に関する調査・試験について，それに係る有効性に関する検討事項，目的，根拠等について記載すること。なお，有効性に関する調査・試験が複数ある場合には，それぞれ必要な数だけ欄を増やして記載すること。
- ○ 有効性に関する調査・試験がある場合には，その実施計画書を製造販売後調査等実施計画書として提出すること。

6.「リスク最小化計画の概要」について

- ○「追加のリスク最小化活動」について，それに係る安全性検討事項，目的，根拠等について記載すること。追加のリスク最小化活動が複数ある場合には，それぞれ必要な数だけ欄を増やして記載すること。

7.「医薬品安全性監視計画，有効性に関する調査・試験の計画及びリスク最小化計画の一覧」について

- ○ それぞれについて，実施中のものだけでなく，予定のものを含めて一覧を作成すること。
- ○ 実施状況欄は，医薬品リスク管理計画の改訂時に，その時点の医薬品リスク管理計画の実施状況について記載すること。

marketing situation, and try to simplify statements by, as appropriate, attaching related data, literature, and any other relevant information to the Form for the purpose of quotation. When a Risk Management Plan is to be submitted as the data required for approval application, pay careful attention to consistency with the related matters of the Common Technical Document.
- ○ When there is more than one "Efficacy-Related Issue", increase the number of columns to the required level and indicate all such issues. When there is no matter to be indicated, it is unnecessary to fill in this subsection.
- ○ When pharmacovigilance activities, implementation of a survey/trial on efficacy, or risk minimization activities are based on the conditions for approval, instructions made by the Pharmaceutical Affairs and Food Sanitation Council, or any other relevant factors, indicate that fact.

4. Section "Overview of Pharmacovigilance Plan"

- ○ As for additional pharmacovigilance activities, indicate Safety Specification related to the activity concerned as well as the objective(s), rationale, and any other relevant aspects of that activity. When there is more than one "additional pharmacovigilance activity", increase the number of columns to the required level and state relevant information on all such activities.
- ○ When there exists any additional pharmacovigilance activity, submit an implementation plan for the activity concerned as an implementation plan for post-marketing surveys, etc.

5. Section "Overview of Plan for Survey/Trial on Efficacy"

- ○ As for survey(s)/trial(s) on efficacy, indicate efficacy-related issues relating to the survey/trial concerned as well as the objective(s), rationale, and any other relevant aspects of that survey/trial. When there is more than one survey/trial on efficacy, increase the number of columns to the required level and state relevant information on all such surveys/trials.
- ○ When there exists any survey/trial on efficacy, submit an implementation plan for the survey/trial on efficacy as an implementation plan for post-marketing surveys, etc.

6. Section "Overview of Risk Minimization Plan"

- ○ As for "additional risk minimization activities", indicate Safety Specification related to the activity concerned as well as the objective(s), rationale, and any other relevant aspects of that activity. When there is more than one "additional risk minimization activity", increase the number of columns to the required level and state relevant information on all such activities.

7. Section "At-a-Glance Tables for Pharmacovigilance Plan, Plan for Survey/Trial on Efficacy, and Risk Minimization Plan"

- ○ In each of the Tables, indicate not only those which are ongoing but also those which are planned to be conducted.
- ○ In the column "Status of implementation", indicate the status of implementation of a Risk Management Plan at the time of its revision.

8.「医薬品リスク管理計画のための組織体制」について

○「責任者」については，安全管理責任者及び製造販売後調査等管理責任者を記載し，兼務の場合はその旨を記載すること。

○「安全管理業務のための組織体制」及び「製造販売後調査等業務のための組織体制」については，製造販売業者におけるそれぞれの業務の全般を概説し，関連する部門について，会社組織全体の中における位置付け及び医薬品リスク管理計画の実施における連携を確認できる組織図等の資料を添付すること。

○「6.2 安全管理業務のための組織体制」において，医薬品リスク管理計画書の作成者を明記すること。

9.「参考資料」について

○ 本計画書に添付する参考資料について，一覧を作成すること。

○ 参考資料として，承認申請に際し申請書に添付した資料の概要(薬事・食品衛生審議会担当部会用)，審査報告書，薬事・食品衛生審議会の審議結果報告書，添付文書(案)を添付すること。

8. Section "Organizational System for Risk Management Plan"

- ○ As for the responsible persons, indicate a safety management supervisor and a supervisor of post-marketing surveys, etc. When a single person holds these two posts, indicate that fact.
- ○ As for "Organizational System for Fulfilling Safety Management Duties" and "Organizational System for Fulfilling Duties Involved in Post-Marketing Surveys, etc.", provide an overview of the individual duties at the MAH concerned, and attach organizational charts or any other relevant documents identifying the following: how functions engaged in these duties are positioned within the entire corporation, and how these functions collaborate with one another in implementing a Risk Management Plan.
- ○ In the subsection "6.2 Organizational System for Fulfilling Safety Management Duties", identify a person who develops a Risk Management Plan.

9. Section "Reference Data"

- ○ Provide a list of reference data to be attached to a Risk Management Plan.
- ○ As reference data, attach the following: summary of data attached to an application document at the time of submission of approval application (for use in the responsible division of the Pharmaceutical Affairs and Food Sanitation Council), review reports, reports of results of review by the Pharmaceutical Affairs and Food Sanitation Council, and draft package insert or prescribing information.

(別添)

1. 使用成績調査実施計画書

(1) 調査の目的(承認条件等の場合には,その旨を記載する。)
(2) 安全性検討事項
(3) 調査の実施計画(案)
　　ア　調査を予定する症例数及び設定根拠
　　イ　調査の対象となる患者(承認に係る効能,効果及び用法,用量に従って当該医薬品を使用する患者)
　　ウ　調査を予定する診療科別の施設数
　　エ　調査の方法
　　オ　調査の実施予定期間
　　カ　調査を行う事項等
　　　　(ア)調査を行う事項
　　　　(イ)重点調査事項,設定根拠及び具体的調査方法
　　キ　解析を行う項目及び方法
　　ク　調査実施のための組織体制(医薬品リスク管理計画書と同じ場合はその旨を記載する。)
　　ケ　調査に係る業務の一部を委託する場合にあっては,当該業務を受託した者の氏名,住所及び当該委託した業務の範囲
(4) 調査の結果に基づいて実施される可能性のある追加の措置及びその開始の決定基準
(5) 調査の実施状況及び得られた結果の評価,又は総合機構への報告を行う節目となる予定の時期及び師の根拠
(6) その他必要な事項

○ 参考資料
　　ア．契約の文書(案)
　　イ．使用成績調査実施要綱(案)
　　ウ．使用成績調査登録票(案)
　　エ．使用成績調査調査票(案)

2. 特定使用成績調査実施計画書

(1) 調査の目的(承認条件等の場合には,その旨を記載する)

(Annex)

1. Protocol of Drug Use Results Survey

    (1) Objective(s) of the survey (When the survey is to be performed in accordance with the conditions for approval of the drug concerned, indicate that fact.)

    (2) Safety Specification

    (3) Protocol (draft) of the survey

        A. The anticipated number of subjects to be included in the survey and the rationale for setting this number

        B. Patients to be included in the survey (i.e. patients who will use the drug concerned in accordance with the approved indication(s) as well as dosage and administration for that drug)

        C. The number of institutions, broken down according to department, which are expected to perform the survey

        D. Methods of the survey

        E. Expected period of the survey

        F. Matters to be surveyed and other information

            A) Matters to be surveyed

            B) Matters subject to intensive survey, rationale for setting the matters, and specific methods for survey

        G. Items to be analyzed and analytical methods

        H. Organizational system for conducting the survey (When this system is the same as that for a Risk Management Plan, indicate that fact.)

        I. When a part of the duties related to the survey is outsourced under contract to another person or organization, indicate the name and address of the contractor as well as the scope of the duties outsourced.

    (4) Possible additional actions to be taken on the basis of results of the survey, and the decision criteria for initiating these actions

    (5) Milestones for evaluating the implementation status of the survey and the results obtained from the survey, or for reporting them to the PMDA, and the rationale for these milestones

    (6) Any other necessary information

○ Reference Data

    A. Agreement document (draft)

    B. Guiding principle for implementation of drug use results survey (draft)

    C. Registration sheet for drug use results survey (draft)

    D. Case report form for drug use results survey (draft)

2. Protocol for Specified Drug Use Survey

    (1) Objective(s) of the survey (When the survey is to be performed in accordance with the conditions

(2)安全性検討事項
(3)調査の実施計画(案)
　　ア　調査を予定する症例数及び設定根拠
　　イ　調査の対象となる患者
　　ウ　調査を予定する診療科別の施設数
　　エ　調査の方法
　　オ　調査の実施予定期間
　　カ　調査を行う事項
　　キ　解析を行う項目及び方法
　　ク　調査実施のための組織体制(医薬品リスク管理計画書と同じ場合はその旨を記載する。)
　　ケ　調査に係る業務の一部を委託する場合にあっては，当該業務を受託した者の氏名，住所及び当該委託した業務の範囲
(4)調査の結果に基づいて実施される可能性のある追加の措置及びその開始の決定基準
(5)調査の実施状況及び得られた結果の評価，又は総合機構への報告を行う節目となる予定の時期及びその根拠
(6)その他必要な事項

○ 参考資料
　　ア．契約の文書(案)
　　イ．特定使用成績調査実施要綱(案)
　　ウ．特定使用成績調査登録票(案)
　　エ．特定使用成績調査調査票(案)

3. 製造販売後臨床試験実施計画書

(1)試験の目的(承認条件等の場合には，その旨を記載する。)
(2)安全性検討事項
(3)試験の実施計画(案)
　　ア　製造販売後臨床試験の依頼をしようとする者の氏名及び住所
　　イ　試験に係る業務の一部を委託する場合にあっては，当該業務を受託した者の氏名，住所及び当該委託した業務の範囲
　　ウ　実施医療機関の名称及び所在地(試験を予定する診療科別の施設数)
　　エ　製造販売後臨床試験責任医師となるべき者の氏名及び職名
　　オ　被験薬の概要
　　カ　試験の方法

for approval of the drug concerned, indicate that fact.)
(2) Safety Specification
(3) Protocol (draft) of the survey
  A. The anticipated number of subjects to be included in the survey and the rationale for setting this number
  B. Patients to be included in the survey
  C. The number of institutions, broken down according to department, which are expected to perform the survey
  D. Methods of the survey
  E. Expected period of the survey
  F. Matters to be surveyed
  G. Items to be analyzed and analytical methods
  H. Organizational system for conducting the survey (When this system is the same as that for a Risk Management Plan, indicate that fact.)
  I. When a part of the duties related to the survey is outsourced under contract to another person or organization, indicate the name and address of the contractor as well as the scope of the duties outsourced.
(4) Possible additional actions to be taken on the basis of results of the survey, and the decision criteria for initiating these actions
(5) Milestone for evaluating the implementation status of the survey and the results obtained from the survey, or for reporting them to the PMDA, and the rationale for these milestones
(6) Any other necessary information

○ Reference Data
  A. Agreement document (draft)
  B. Guiding principle for implementation of specified drug use survey (draft)
  C. Registration sheet for specified drug use survey (draft)
  D. Case report form for specified drug use survey (draft)

3. Protocol for Post-Marketing Clinical Study

(1) Objective(s) of the study (When the study is to be performed in accordance with the conditions for approval of the drug concerned, indicate that fact.)
(2) Safety Specification
(3) Protocol (draft) for the study
  A. The name and address of the person who intends to sponsor the post-marketing clinical study
  B. When a part of the duties involved in the study is outsourced under contract to another person or organization, indicate the name and address of the contractor as well as the scope of the duties outsourced.
  C. The name and address of each medical institution participating in the study (together with

キ 被験者の選定に関する事項(試験の対象患者)
ク 試験を予定する症例数及び設定根拠
ケ 観察項目及び評価項目等の調査を行う事項
コ 試験の実施予定期間
サ 解析を行う項目及び方法
シ 原資料の閲覧に関する事項
ス 記録(データを含む。)の保存に関する事項
セ 製造販売後臨床試験調整医師に委嘱した場合にあっては,その氏名及び職名
ソ 製造販売後臨床試験調整委員会に委嘱した場合にあっては,これを構成する医師等の氏名及び職名
タ 効果安全性評価委員会を設置したときは,その旨
チ 製造販売後臨床試験の依頼をしようとする者は,当該製造販売後臨床試験が被験者に対して製造販売後臨床試験薬が効果を有しないこと,及び当該製造販売後臨床試験への参加についてあらかじめ文書による説明と同意を得ることが困難な者を対象にすることが予測される場合には,その旨及び次に掲げる事項
　(ア)当該製造販売後臨床試験が,試験への参加についてあらかじめ文書による説明と同意を得ることが困難と予測される者を対象にしなければならないことの説明
　(イ)当該製造販売後臨床試験において,予測される被験者への不利益が必要な最小限度のものであることの説明
ツ 製造販売後臨床試験を依頼しようとする者は,当該製造販売後臨床試験が,試験への参加についてあらかじめ文書による説明と同意及び代諾者の同意を得ることが困難と予測される者を対象にしている場合には,その旨及び次に掲げる事項
　(ア)現在における治療方法では被験者となるべき者に対して十分な効果が期待できないことの説明
　(イ)被験薬の使用により被験者となるべき者の生命の危険が回避できる可能性が十分にあることの説明
　(ウ)効果安全性評価委員会が設置されている旨
テ 試験実施のための組織体制(医薬品リスク管理計画書と同じ場合はその旨を記載する。)

(4)試験の結果に基づいて実施される可能性のある追加の措置及びその開始の決定基準
(5)試験の実施状況及び得られた結果の評価,又は総合機構への報告を行う節目となる予定の時期及びその根拠
(6)その他必要な事項

○ 参考資料
　ア．契約の文書(案)
　イ．被験者に対して行う説明文書(案)及び同意文書(案)
　ウ．製造販売後臨床試験登録票(案)
　エ．症例報告書(案)

the expected number of institutions, broken down according to department, which are expected to perform the trial)

D. The name(s) and job title(s) of the person(s) to be appointed as post-marketing clinical study investigator(s)

E. Overview of the test drug

F. Methods of the study

G. Description of subject selection (for those who will be included in the study)

H. The anticipated number of subjects to be included in the study and the rationale for setting this number

I. Items to be surveyed, including observation items, evaluation items and any other relevant investigation items

J. Expected period of the study

K. Items to be analyzed and analytical methods

L. Description of direct access to source documents

M. Description of record (including data) keeping

N. When a coordinating investigator of the post-marketing clinical study is designated and entrusted with the responsibility for the coordination of investigators at different participating institutions, indicate the name and job tile of the coordinating investigator.

O. When a coordinating committee of the post-marketing clinical study is established and entrusted with the responsibility for the coordination of conduct of the study, indicate the names and job titles of medical doctors and other persons who constitute the committee.

P. When a Data and Safety Monitoring Board is established, indicate that fact.

Q. The person who intends to sponsor a post-marketing clinical study shall state in the protocol, if applicable, that the post-marketing study drug affords no intended clinical benefit to the subject, and that some subjects are to be enrolled in the clinical study although it would be difficult to explain in writing the study-related information to them prior to study initiation and obtain their written, prior consent to participate in the study. The protocol shall also include the following information:

(A) Reasons why some subjects are to be enrolled in the post-marketing clinical study concerned, although it would be difficult to explain in writing the study-related information to them prior to study initiation and obtain their written, prior consent to participate in the study

(B) Explanation that the potential disadvantages which the subject may incur in the post-marketing clinical study concerned are minimized

R. The person who intends to sponsor a post-marketing clinical study shall state in the protocol that, if applicable, some subjects are to be enrolled in the post-marketing clinical study concerned although it would be difficult to explain in writing the study-related information to them prior to study initiation and obtain their written, prior consent to participate in the study, and to obtain informed consent from their legally acceptable representatives. The protocol shall also include the following information:

(A) Explanation that currently available treatments are unlikely to achieve sufficient therapeutic effects in the prospective subject

(B) Explanation that there is a sufficient possibility of saving the life of the prospective subject by using the test drug

(C) A note that a Data and Safety Monitoring Board has been established for the study concerned

S. Organization system for conducting the study (When this system is the same as that for a Risk Management Plan, indicate that fact.)

(4) Possible additional actions to be taken on the basis of results of the study, and the decision criteria for initiating these actions

(5) Milestones for evaluating the implementation status of the study and the results obtained from the study, or for reporting them to the PMDA, and the rationale for these milestones

(6) Any other necessary information

○ Reference Data
  A. Agreement document (draft)
  B. Written information given to the study subject (draft) and informed consent form (draft)
  C. Registration sheet for post-marketing clinical study (draft)
  D. Case Report Form (draft)

薬害に関する公的教育について

2010年に公表された薬害肝炎に関する最終提言をきっかけとして、日本においては薬害を教育の中に取り込む動きが始まりました。ここでは二つの動きについて紹介します。

1. （社）日本薬学会と文部科学省の取り組み

日本薬学会と文部科学省は専門委員会を設置して、薬学教育モデルコアカリキュラム改訂の検討を行っています。このコアカリキュラムの趣旨は次のとおりです。

> 近年、医療技術や医薬品の創製・適用に大きな科学的進歩が達成されました。そこで、医療を担う主役の一人である薬剤師にも、最先端の知識と研究能力が求められるようになってきました。これが薬剤師教育に6年制課程が導入された理由です。（中略）これまでの知識教育に偏ったカリキュラムではなく、知識教育、技能教育、態度教育を組み込んだ統合的なカリキュラムが求められたのです。
>
> これから示します「薬学教育モデルコアカリキュラム」は、日本私立薬科大学協会と国公立大学薬学部長会からの案を統合して2002年に組まれ、「実務実習モデルコアカリキュラム」と「卒業実習カリキュラム」を加えて2003年に完成したものです。

2013年2月に公表されたコアカリキュラム改訂案の薬害教育に関するポイントは以下の通りです。コアカリキュラムは最終的に、平成25年度に決定し、26年度または27年から開始予定になっています。

A 基本事項
(1) 省略
(2) 医療安全と薬害の防止
　1. 医薬品に関わるリスクマネジメントにおいて薬剤師の責任と義務を説明できる。
　2. 医薬品が関わる代表的な医療過誤やインシデントの事例を列挙し、その原因と防止策を説明できる。
　3. 医薬品が関わる薬害の例（サリドマイド、スモン、非加熱血液製剤、ソリブジンなど）についてその原因と社会的背景を説明できる。
　4. 代表的な薬害や重篤な副作用の例について、これらを回避するための手段を討議する（態度）。

Public Education of Drug-Induced Suffering

The final proposal regarding drug-induced hepatitis published in 2010 triggered promotion of movement toward incorporation of drug-induced suffering into education in Japan. Two activities are introduced in this section.

1. Activities by the Pharmaceutical Society of Japan, a public interest incorporated association, and the Ministry of Education, Culture, Sports, Science and Technology (MEXT)

The Pharmaceutical Society of Japan and the MEXT have established an experts council to discuss revision of the Pharmaceutical Education Model Core Curriculum. The objective of this Core Curriculum is as stated below.

> *A great deal of scientific advancement has recently been achieved in medical technologies as well as drug discovery and application. Along with the advancement, pharmacists, one of the main players in the healthcare field, need to acquire leading-edge knowledge and research capabilities. For this reason, a 6-year course was introduced for training pharmacists in pharmaceutical schools.*

The Objective continues:

> *... The past curriculum placed an overemphasis on knowledge, while what was needed instead was an integrated curriculum incorporating knowledge, skill, and attitude into pharmacopedics.*
> *The "Pharmaceutical Education Model Core Curriculum" introduced below was completed in 2003 by adding the "Practical On-Site Training Curriculum" and the "Graduation Training Curriculum" to a merger in 2002 of the proposals made by the Association of Private Pharmaceutical Schools of Japan and those made by the Committee of Directors of Departments of Pharmaceutical Sciences at National and Public Universities.*

The important points regarding education of drug-induced suffering in the revised Core Curriculum that was published in February 2013 are described below. This Core Curriculum is to be finalized in the academic year 2013 and will start in the academic year 2014 or 2015.

A Basic Matters
(1) Omission

(2) Safety in healthcare and prevention of drug-induced suffering
  1. Be able to explain the responsibilities and obligations of pharmacists in risk management involving drugs.
  2. Be able to list representative medical malpractices and incidents involving drugs, and explain their causes and preventive measures.
  3. Be able to explain causes of and social background for incidents of drug-induced suffering (e.g. thalidomide, SMON, non-heated blood products, and sorivudine).
  4. Regarding typical cases of drug-induced suffering and serious adverse drug reactions, discuss

(3) 省略

2. 厚生労働省の取り組み

　厚生労働省では文部科学省の協力を得て，中学3年生を対象とした薬害を学ぶための教材「薬害を学ぼう」を作成し，2011年4月より全国の中学校に配布しています。この教材は主に社会科における消費者の保護に関連する内容です。医薬品による薬害を知るとともに，その発生の過程や社会的な動き等を学ぶことを通じて，今後，同様の被害が起こらない社会の仕組みの在り方などを考えることを目的とするものです。

教材の概略は次の通りです。
・薬害ってなんだろう(薬害事件と年表のイラスト)。ここではジフテリア予防接種事件，スモン事件，サリドマイド事件，筋短縮症事件，HIV感染事件，HCV感染事件，MMRワクチン事件，陣痛促進剤事件，CJD事件が年表に取り上げられています。
・薬害による被害者の声(証言)の紹介。
・ワークシートによる学習のポイント
　　①なぜ薬害は起こったのだろう？(スモン事件とサリドマイド事件の被害者の証言事例として)
　　②各関係者の社会における役割について(国/PMDA，製薬会社，国民(消費者)，医療従事者(医療機関)/薬局)
　　③薬害発生を防ぐために各関係者の立場で行うこと(国/PMDA，製薬会社，国民(消費者)，医療従事者(医療機関)/薬局)
　　④薬害が起こらない社会にするために，社会をどのような仕組みに変えなければならないか？

　厚生労働省では，「薬害を学び再発を防止するための教育に関する検討会」を設置し，2012年10月には11回目の検討会を行いました。これらの結果，2012年3月に行われた調査では，全国11,170校の中学校のうち，21.9％に当たる2448校でこの教材が使われていました。今後の一層の浸透が期待されています。

measures of prevention (attitude).

(3) Omission

2. Activities by the Ministry of Health, Labour and Welfare (MHLW)

The MHLW, in cooperation with the MEXT, prepared teaching material entitled "Let's learn about drug-induced suffering!" for third-grade junior high school students to study drug-induced suffering, and have distributed it to junior high schools throughout Japan since April 2011. This teaching material is primarily concerned with protection of consumers in school classes of social studies. Its objectives are to raise students' awareness of drug-induced suffering, learn the development process of drug-induced suffering, social responses to such development, and any other relevant matters, through which students are encouraged to consider the social framework preventing occurrences of similar types of health damage to those in the past.

The contents of this teaching material are outlined below.
- What is drug-induced suffering? (A chronological table of the past incidents of drug-induced suffering and illustrations are presented.) This chronological table includes the diphtheria immunization incident, the SMON incident, the thalidomide incident, the muscle contracture incident, the HIV infection incident, the HCV infection incident, the MMR vaccine incident, the labor-inducing drugs incident, and the CJD incident.
- Introduction of voices (testimonies) of victims of drug-induced suffering
- Key points for learning through the use of worksheet
    (1) Why did drug-induced suffering occur? (using testimonies of victims of the SMON incident and the thalidomide incident as case studies)
    (2) Roles of those concerned in society (the national government/the Pharmaceuticals and Medical Devices Agency (PMDA), pharmaceutical companies, the general public (consumers), and healthcare professionals (medical institutions)/pharmacies)
    (3) What those concerned should do individually to prevent the occurrence of drug-induced suffering (the national government/the PMDA, pharmaceutical companies, the general public (consumers), and healthcare professionals (medical institutions)/pharmacies)
    (4) How shall we change a social framework so as to create a society in which no drug-induced suffering will occur?

The MHLW has established the "Administrative Committee on Education with the Aim of Learning and Preventing Drug-Induced Suffering" and held the 11th meeting of the Committee in October 2012. As a result of the efforts by the Committee, the survey in March 2012 revealed that out of a total of 11,170 junior high schools in Japan, 2,448 (21.9%) schools used this teaching material. It is expected that an increasing number of junior high schools will use it in the future.

全国薬害被害者団体連絡協議会

　全国薬害被害者団体連絡協議会は，主として第2章で取り上げた薬害事件の被害者がそれぞれ結成した団体が協議会として1999年に結成されました。加入している諸団体は次の11団体です。

- サリドマイド福祉センター
- イレッサ薬害被害者の会
- MMR被害児を救援する会
- 大阪HIV薬害訴訟原告団
- 東京HIV訴訟原告団
- スモンの会全国連絡協議会
- 京都スモン基金
- 薬害ヤコブ病被害者・弁護団全国連絡会議
- 陣痛促進剤による被害を考える会
- 薬害筋短縮症の会
- 薬害肝炎訴訟原告団

　この連絡協議会としての活動は大きく分けて次の二つです。

1) 薬害根絶フォーラム
　このフォーラムは1999年より毎年秋に行われています。薬害被害の実態としてノンフィクション映画の上映や，被害者による講演，討論を各地で開催しています。このフォーラムは一般市民や専門家に公開されています。

2) 薬害根絶デー
　連絡協議会は1999年8月24日に厚生労働省敷地内に「薬害根絶誓いの碑」が建立されたことから，8月24日を薬害根絶デーと定めて，毎年，厚生労働大臣の出席を求めて行政との話し合いを行い，また行政への要望書を提出しています。

　2012年の根絶デーにおいて厚生労働大臣に提出された要望書の主な要点は以下の通りです。
- 2012年の薬害根絶デーに大臣が参加すること。
- 小・中・高の公的教育において2011年から配布された薬害教育の教材を活用すること。学習指導要領に薬害を記載すること。副作用被害救済制度を周知すること。
- 高等専門教育において薬害教育プログラムの実施率を高めること。

Japanese National Liaison Council for Associations of Victims of Drug-Induced Suffering

In 1999, the Japanese National Liaison Council for Associations of Victims of Drug-Induced Suffering (hereinafter referred to as the National Liaison Council) was established primarily by the associations organized by victims of the individual incidents of drug-induced suffering described in Chapter 2. Eleven associations listed below join this Council.

- Thalidomide Welfare Center
- Association of Victims of Iressa-Induced Suffering
- Association for Relief of MMR Victim Children
- Osaka Drug-Induced HIV Lawsuit Plaintiff Group
- Tokyo HIV Lawsuit Plaintiff Group
- Nationwide Liaison Council for Associations of SMON victims
- Kyoto SMON Fund
- Nationwide Liaison Council for Drug-Induced CJD Victims and Litigation Lawyers Group
- Association for Study of Health Damage Caused by Labor-Inducing Drugs
- Association of Drug-Induced Muscle Contracture
- Drug-Induced Hepatitis Lawsuit Plaintiff Group

The National Liaison Council holds major two activities as described below.

1) Forum for Eradication of Drug-Induced Suffering
This forum is held in autumn every year since 1999. For the purpose of communicating the actual situation of victims of drug-induced suffering, non-fiction movies are shown, victims as speakers give talks to the audience, and discussion is held. This forum is conducted at different places in Japan, and open to the general public and to specialists.

2) Day for Eradication of Drug-Induced Suffering
On August 24, 1999, the "Monument of Oath for Eradication of Drug-Induced Suffering" was built in the premises of the Ministry of Health, Labour and Welfare. The National Liaison Council therefore designates August 24 as the Day for Eradication of Drug-Induced Suffering. On this day every year, the National Liaison Council holds meetings with the administration which the Council asks the Minister of Health, Labour and Welfare to attend, and submits written request to the administration.

On the Day for Eradication of Drug-Induced Suffering in 2012, the written request submitted to the Minister of Health, Labour and Welfare contained the major points as listed below.
- Participation of the Minister of Health, Labour and Welfare in the 2012 Day for Eradication of Drug-Induced Suffering
- In the public education at elementary, junior high, and high schools, utilization of the teaching material regarding

・厚生労働省では実施しているが，文部科学省においても医学，歯学，薬学教育の問題を議論する審議会，検討会の委員として被害者の参加を促すこと。
・医学生，医療従事者による被害者に対する誹謗中傷のインターネット書き込みが見られることに対して，具体的な人権教育を推進すること。
・モデル・コア・カリキュラムに関する要望。
・その他生涯学習に薬害を取り入れることの推進など。

drug-induced suffering that was distributed starting in 2011. Inclusion of education on drug-induced suffering in the Japanese state government determined guidelines for teaching at elementary, junior high, and high schools. Increase of the public's awareness of the Relief System for Adverse Drug Reactions.
・ Increase of implementation rates for education programs on drug-induced suffering at higher specialized education
・ The Ministry of Education, Culture, Sports, Science and Technology should encourage victims to participate in, as members, meetings of advisory councils and study groups which discuss education-related issues in the fields of medical science, dentistry, and pharmaceutical science, as the Ministry of Health, Labour and Welfare has already promoted such efforts.
・ Promotion of specific human-rights education in response to the fact that some students at medical schools and healthcare professionals have allegedly written slanders and libels against victims on the internet
・ Request regarding "Model Core Curriculum"
・ Others, including promotion of incorporation of drug-induced suffering into life-long learning

承認条件

　開発段階で得られる有効性・安全性に関する知見は，極めて限定的なものであることは言うまでもありません。治験では対象となる患者の数は限られており，その年齢構成，性別，併用薬，合併症等に厳しい制限があります。さらには，投与期間も限られており，有効性の評価も，臨床検査値等の代替指標が用いられることも多く，延命効果等の真の指標への効果が分からない場合が多々あります。また，治験を行う医師や医療機関は，当該新薬や疾病についての専門的な知識と経験を有する等の点で，実際の医療の場とは大きく環境が異なります。

　しかしながら，開発段階でより幅広く，多数の患者を対象とした臨床試験を義務付けることは，開発・審査段階での情報の質と量は高まりますが，開発段階の負荷も高まることから，開発の遅延につながる可能性が大きく，開発が断念される場合も増えると考えられます。

　日本では世界に先駆けて昭和35年に制定された薬事法の中に「承認条件」の規定が設けられており（法律第145号），開発段階で安全性等に関する情報が特に限られている医薬品や承認後の安全性確保が特に必要な医薬品については，承認条件が付された上で承認されることになっています。

■薬事法第79条の規定
・承認には条件または期間を付し，また，これを変更することが出来る
・承認の条件または期間は，保健衛生上の危害の発生を防止するため必要な最小限度のものに限る
・条件や期間は承認を受ける者に対し不当な義務を課すものであってはならない
・条件を守らない場合には承認の取り消し，一部変更などを命ずることが出来る（2002年の薬事法改正による追加）

　承認条件には大きく分けて，①承認後一定期間または一定数に達するまで医薬品を使用した患者のすべての情報の収集を義務付けるもの（全例調査），②承認後追加的な臨床試験の実施を義務付けるもの（市販後臨床試験），③承認後一定期間，医薬品を使用できる医療機関または医師を限定するもの（使用限定）があります。

　この承認条件は，開発・審査段階で把握されたリスク要因に対して承認後にリスクの最小化と重点的な安全性監視を行うという，リスク管理計画の一部をなすものになります。従来は承認条件において，どのようなリスク要因に対して承認条件を付したのかが明確に示されないことが

Conditional Approval System

It is needless to say that information and knowledge on efficacy and safety of a drug obtained during its development phase is extremely limited. In clinical trials, the number of patients enrolled is limited and firm restrictions are imposed on the demographic factors of eligible patients which include, among others, age, gender, medications of concomitant use, and complications. Treatment period is also limited. Efficacy evaluation frequently uses surrogate variables such as clinical laboratory tests, and for this reason, effectiveness of a particular drug on the true variable, e.g. life-prolonging effect, cannot be identified in many cases. In addition, physicians and medical institutions participating in clinical trials possess specialized knowledge and experience regarding the new drug and disease(s) under evaluation and in this respect, they are substantially different from those at actual medical sites.

On the other hand, making it obligatory to perform clinical studies covering a wider range of and a greater number of patients in the development phase would improve the quality and quantity of information available at the stages of development and approval review and at the same time, increase burdens imposed during the development phase. This may highly likely delay development and even worse, could result in some development projects being abandoned.

In Japan, the Pharmaceutical Affairs Law (PAL) established in 1960 (Law No. 145) specifies the provisions regarding "Conditions for License, etc."; regarding new drug products for which information on safety, etc. obtained in the development phase is limited or post-approval risk minimization measures are particularly required, they shall be approved with the condition(s) for approval attached. Japan was an international pioneer in establishing such a conditional approval system.

■ Provisions in Article 79 of the PAL
- Conditions or expiration dates may be attached to the approval, and may be subject to change.
- The conditions or expiration dates attached to the approval shall be confined to the necessary minimum to prevent occurrence of hazards to public health and hygiene.
- The conditions or expiration dates attached to the approval shall not impose unreasonable obligations on persons intending to obtain approval.
- The Minister of Health, Labour and Welfare is entitled to cancel the approval or order changes in part of the approval when the person granted it has violated the condition(s) attached to it. (This provision was added when the PAL was revised in 2002.)

There are three major conditions as follows: (1) a condition that makes it obligatory to collect information on all patients using the drug for a fixed period after approval or until a certain number of patients is reached (all-patient post-marketing surveillance); (2) a condition that makes it obligatory to perform additional clinical studies after approval (post-marketing clinical study); and (3) a condition that makes it obligatory to restrict use of the drug by limiting the number of medical institutions or physicians that can access the drug for a fixed period after approval (restricted access).

多かったのですが，今後はリスク管理計画の導入により，目的・手段等がより詳細に定められるものと期待されます。

承認条件による効果としては，安全性の向上，開発期間の短縮等があげられます。

安全性の向上
①長期投与における安全性の確認や副作用発生率の把握：臨床試験段階では投与期間は限られているため，長期投与による副作用を把握しにくいのですが，承認後は長期投与が行われる可能性があります。承認条件の付与により特定の副作用に注目して副作用の発生率の把握や，臨床試験段階と実際の医療の場で使われた場合との副作用発生率の変化等の把握が可能となります。
②小児等の特殊な患者群における安全性の確認： 臨床試験段階では，基本的には小児や高齢者，肝機能や腎機能等に障害のある患者，妊娠中の女性等のいわゆる特殊な患者群は治験の対象から外されることが多くみられます。しかし，実際の医療の場では治験段階で検討されなかった患者にも投薬される可能性があり，そのような事例を注意深く集めて解析することで貴重な情報を得ることができます。その結果は，医療の現場にフィードバックされ，安全な使用が可能となります。
③特に全例調査などが指示された場合，企業に対しては医薬品の納入について，また医療機関や医師に対しては使用について，それぞれ慎重な姿勢で臨むことを求める行政の意思表示となり，安全対策への注意喚起につながります。

有効性の向上
①長期投与による真のエンドポイントに対する有効性の確認：多くの場合，臨床試験においては，代替指標を用いて，新薬の有効性は評価されますが，延命効果等の真の指標に対する効果は，市販後における薬剤疫学的な追跡によらなければ把握できません。抗がん剤についても，以前は，がんの縮小という代替指標で効果が評価されていたのですが，現在は，治験段階においても延命効果という真の指標で評価されるようになってきました。
②小児等の特殊な患者群に対する有効性の確認：安全性と同様に，特殊な患者群に対する有効性も，承認後に把握することが可能となります。

The conditions for approval constitute part of the Risk Management Plan with which post-marketing risk minimization and intensive pharmacovigilance is performed on risk factors that have been identified in the development and approval review phases. Conventionally, it has not been frequently clarified which risk factors of a particular drug required conditions for approval attached to it. From now on, however, introduction of the Risk Management Plan scheme is expected to determine objectives, procedures, and other relevant matters in more detail.

The effects of the conditional approval system include, among others, improvement of safety and shortening of development period.

Improvement of safety
(1) Confirmation of safety and of incidence rates of adverse drug reactions (ADRs) during long-term treatment: In the clinical trial phase, treatment periods are limited and it is therefore difficult to identify ADRs related to long-term treatment. In the post-marketing phase, however, long-term treatment may be administered in actual clinical settings. Attachment of conditions of approval enables determination of incidence rates of particular ADRs of interest, which makes it possible to understand differences in the incidence rates of such ADRs between the clinical trial phase and actual clinical settings.
(2) Confirmation of safety in special populations such as pediatric patients: In the clinical trial phase, so-called special populations including, among others, children, geriatric patients, those with hepatic and renal impairment, and pregnant women are in many cases excluded from clinical trials. In actual clinical settings, however, drugs may be administered to patients who have not been evaluated in the clinical trial phase. When data on such unevaluated patients are carefully collected and analyzed in the post-marketing phase, valuable information is obtained. Results of such analysis are fed back to medical sites so as to promote safe use of drugs.
(3) Especially when all-patient post-marketing surveillance is given as an approval condition, this is the explicit representation of the drug administration's intention that they specially require the company concerned to exercise caution upon delivery of the drug to medical institutions and at the same time, medical institutions and physicians to exercise caution upon use of the drug. This leads to alerting toward safety measures.

Improvement of efficacy
(1) Confirmation of efficacy on the true endpoint during long-term treatment: In many clinical trials, efficacy evaluation for new drugs uses surrogate variables. Efficacy on true endpoints, e.g. life-prolonging effect, cannot be identified unless post-marketing pharmacoepidemiologic studies follow up patients. For anticancer agents, for example, tumor size reduction was used as a surrogate variable for efficacy evaluation. At present, however, life-prolonging effect, a true variable, is used for evaluation of efficacy of anticancer agents even in the clinical trial phase.
(2) Confirmation of efficacy in special populations such as pediatric patients: As in the case of safety, the conditional approval system enables confirmation of efficacy of drugs in special populations in the

開発期間の短縮
　①開発段階で行うべき臨床試験等の一部を承認後に実施：臨床試験の一部を必要に応じて市販後に行うことにより，開発期間の短縮等が可能となります．第三相試験を市販後に行うなど，日本人症例が限られたものについて，承認後に日本人症例を集めることにより，開発期間の短縮が可能となります．その分市販後の安全対策に比重をかける必要があります．
　②小児効能等を承認後に追加的に開発：小児の効能は成人の効能と同時に開発されるのが理想ですが，成人に対する効能が確立した後に小児の効能を開発することにより，全体の効率化を図ることができます．
　③稀な副作用の発見のための大規模な治験を承認後の市販後調査で代替：米国では稀な副作用を開発段階で発見するために大規模な治験を要求しているケースがみられますが，市販後における厳密な使用成績調査等を行うことで，開発段階の負荷を軽減するとともに，開発期間の短縮が可能となります．ただし，市販後の使用成績調査は治験に較べてデータの質が劣ること等に注意しなければなりません．

その他の効果
　①全例調査等においては，医療関係者に対して適正使用に必要な情報の徹底が図られる必要があるため，結果的に厳格な管理下で使用されることとなり，市販直後の不適正な使用の防止が期待されます．
　②しかしながら，薬事法には承認条件の付与について制限的な規定が設けられています．無原則的な承認条件の付与は，製薬企業に対して無駄な時間と費用を要求することとなるだけではなく，医療機関に対しても，不必要な時間と労力を要求し，更には，医療の場への新薬の迅速な提供が阻害される恐れがあります．承認条件の付与は基本的には薬の安全性の確保のためであることが，薬事法に規定された趣旨です．

承認条件と全例調査
　1998年3月から2010年7月までの間に承認された新医薬品数と承認条件が付いた品目数，さらに承認条件として全例調査が付与された状況を表に示します．この間承認された新医薬品数は589，承認条件が付いた品目数は193で，全体の33％です．さらに，承認条件のうち全例調査が指示された品目は119で，承認条件付与のうち62％を占めます．しかしこの割合は一定でなく，ある時期を境にして大きく変動しています．2002年にイレッサが承認，発売され，その直後から間質性肺炎などの肺障害が拡大したことは2章で述べたとおりですが，イレッサには全例調査

post-marketing phase.

Shortening of development period

(1) Post-approval implementation of some of the clinical studies that should be conducted in the development phase: When some clinical studies are performed in the post-marketing phase as appropriate, the development period can be shortened. When data on Japanese cases are collected after approval is granted to a particular drug since the scope of Japanese patients treated with the drug is limited, e.g. performing phase III studies in the post-marketing phase, the development period can be shortened. In such case, however, more importance needs to be attached to post-marketing safety measures of the drug.

(2) Post-approval development for pediatric indication: It is ideal to develop a drug with indication(s) simultaneously for pediatric patients and adults. When, for a drug which has already received an official approval for indication(s) in adults, development of the drug for pediatric indication(s) is undertaken, the whole process of development phase can be made more efficient.

(3) Post-marketing surveillance performed in place of large-scale clinical trials to detect rare ADRs: In the US, large-scale clinical trials are sometimes required for the purpose of detecting rare ADRs in the development phase. When strict Drug Use Results Surveys and other relevant surveys of a particular drug are performed in the post-marketing phase, the burdens imposed on the development of the drug can be reduced and at the same time, the development period can be shortened. However, attention should be paid to the fact that data obtained from post-marketing Drug Use Results Surveys are inferior in quality to those obtained from clinical trials.

Other effects

(1) In all-patient post-marketing surveillance, attempts need to be made to fully disseminate information necessary for proper use of drugs to healthcare professionals, resulting in strict control of use of the drug concerned. As a result, prevention of improper use of drugs in the early phase after the start of marketing is expected.

(2) The PAL prescribes the restrictive provisions regarding attachment of conditions to approval. Attachment of approval conditions without any rule to go by may force pharmaceutical companies to waste time and costs, cause medical institutions to spend unnecessary time and labor, and even worse, hamper prompt provision of new drugs to medical care sites. As specified in the PAL, the basic purpose of attaching conditions to approvals is to secure the safety of drugs.

Conditions for approval and all-patient post-marketing surveillance

For a period from March 1998 to July 2010, the number of new drugs approved, the number of drugs for which conditions were attached to their approval, and the number of drugs to which implementation of all-patient post-marketing surveillance was required as a condition for their approval are shown in the table on the following page. During this period, a total of 589 new drugs were approved, and to 193 (33%) out of them, approval conditions were attached. Of the drugs given the approval conditions, all-patient post-marketing surveillance was required for 119 drugs, which accounted for 62% of those given the approval conditions.

表　承認条件と全例調査

承認(年)	承認件数	承認条件付	全例調査付	全例調査の割合(%)
1998年3月から	32	14	5	35.7
1999	61	23	9	39.1
2000	66	14	5	35.7
2001	38	13	3	23.1
2002	39	14	1	7.1
2003	28	12	9	75.0
2004	27	12	7	58.3
2005	31	12	11	91.7
2006	53	12	11	91.7
2007	58	16	14	87.5
2008	54	24	24	100.0
2009	54	13	9	69.2
2010年7月まで	48	14	11	78.6

の承認条件は付きませんでした。このイレッサ事件発生の翌年から，承認条件に占める全例調査の指示の割合は飛躍的に増加しました。明らかにイレッサ事件の影響があったと考えられます。制度があっても適切に運用できるかどうかで，制度の実効性が左右された事例であると考えられます。

Table Approval conditions and all-patient post-marketing surveillance

Year of approval	No. of new drugs approved	Drugs given approval conditions	Drugs given all-patient post-marketing surveillance as an approval condition	Percentage of all-patient post-marketing surveillance (%)
From March 1998	32	14	5	35.7
1999	61	23	9	39.1
2000	66	14	5	35.7
2001	38	13	3	23.1
2002	39	14	1	7.1
2003	28	12	9	75.0
2004	27	12	7	58.3
2005	31	12	11	91.7
2006	53	12	11	91.7
2007	58	16	14	87.5
2008	54	24	24	100.0
2009	54	13	9	69.2
To July 2010	48	14	11	78.6

The percentage of new drugs given a condition of all-patient post-marketing surveillance in the total of those given any approval condition did not remain constant but substantially increased after a certain time. As described in Chapter 2, gefitinib was approved and launched onto the market in 2002, and immediately after that, lung disorders such as interstitial pneumonia occurred and expanded. For gefitinib, implementation of all-patient post-marketing surveillance was not required as a condition for its approval. In the years following the occurrence of the gefitinib incident, the percentage of all-patient post-marketing surveillance in the total of approval conditions began to increase dramatically. It is evident that the gefitinib incident influenced the situation of attachment of approval conditions. This indicates that even if a system is established, its effectiveness is determined by whether or not it is properly administered.

市販直後調査制度

厚労省は，新薬を対象とした市販直後調査制度を2001年10月から実施した。即ち，
①新薬販売開始前後の一定期間製造販売業者等が責任を持って新薬の適正使用情報の徹底を行うこと
②市販直後の期間は安全性情報に特に注意を払うべき期間であり，常に医療機関にリマインドしながら販売するとともに，重篤な副作用等が発生した場合に遅滞なく報告できるよう一定期間はMRが一定の頻度でフォローアップを行うこと
により，適正使用の徹底と，副作用の発生動向を遅れることなく，網羅的に把握できるようにすることを目的としている。

市販直後調査は新薬を対象とし，期間は販売開始後6ヵ月間である。具体的な調査の実施方法は図のとおりである。

なお，市販直後調査期間終了後2ヵ月以内に，市販直後調査実施報告書を市販直後調査計画書と共に提出することとされている。

▶市販直後調査の流れ

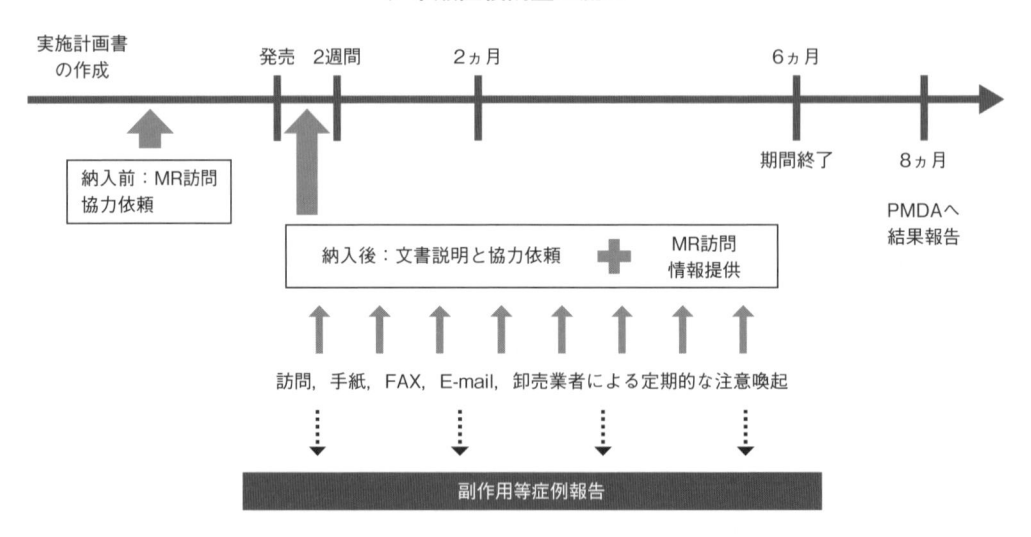

Early Post-marketing Phase Risk Minimization and Vigilance (EPRV) system

The MHLW started the Early Post-marketing Phase Risk Minimization and Vigilance (EPRV) system for new drugs in October 2001. The objectives of this system are to sufficiently communicate information on proper use and to comprehensively determine trends of appearance of ADRs promptly by taking the following measures:

(1) MAH will be responsible for sufficiently communicating information on the proper use of a new drug for a specified period around the start of marketing of a new drug.

(2) The early post-marketing phase is a period when special attention should be given to safety information and the marketing of a new drug should regularly be carried out by stressing that MR should follow up with medical institutions at certain intervals in a predetermined period do that the appearance of serious ADRs, etc. can be reported without delay.

New drugs are subject to EPRV and the duration is 6 months after the start of marketing. With respect to the specific method see **Figure** below.

Reporting on the results to PMDA is required together with the submission of the implementation plan within 2 months after the end of the period.

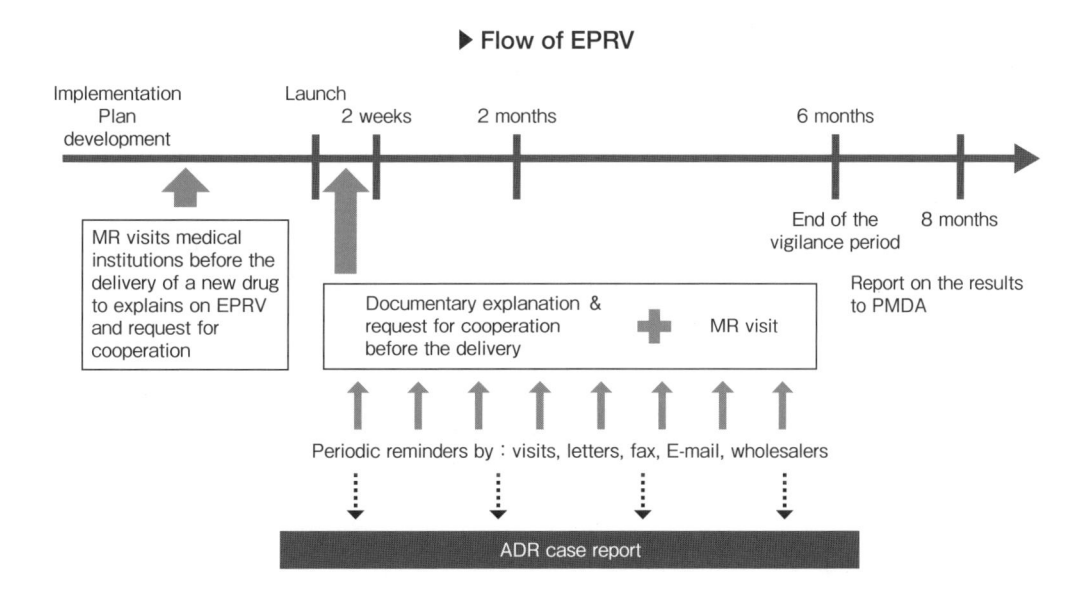

▶ **Flow of EPRV**

医薬品副作用被害救済制度の概要

救済の主な支給要件は以下のとおりである。
① 民事責任の追及が困難な場合,すなわち,本来の医薬品の製造販売業者,販売業者,医療機関等,ほかに損害賠償の責任を有する者の存在が明らかな場合は,対象外である。
② 「適正」に使用されたことが要件で,本来の使用目的とは異なる「不適正目的」や使用上の注意事項に反する「不適正使用」の場合は,対象外である。
③ 医薬品の薬理作用によって生じる有害反応である「副作用」が対象であり,医薬品に細菌やウイルス等が混入したことによる「感染」や異物による汚染は対象外である。
④ 副作用の中でも「入院相当の治療が必要な被害」,「1・2級程度の障害」,「死亡」の場合を対象としており,軽微な副作用は対象外である。
⑤ 「受忍」が適当でない副作用を対象としている。すなわち,「重い」副作用があっても使用が必要な抗がん剤等の医薬品(除外医薬品)による副作用,救命のためやむを得ず通常の使用量を越えて医薬品を使用したことによる副作用等,本来の治療のため受忍を求めることが適当と考えられる副作用は対象外であり,「除外医薬品」としては,抗がん剤,免疫抑制剤等が指定されている。

制度の概要は図のとおりである。給付の請求には,副作用の治療を行った医師の診断書や投薬証明書が必要となるので,請求者は医師の協力を得る必要がある。

▶ **給付の請求から給付の決定まで**(総合機構ホームページ)

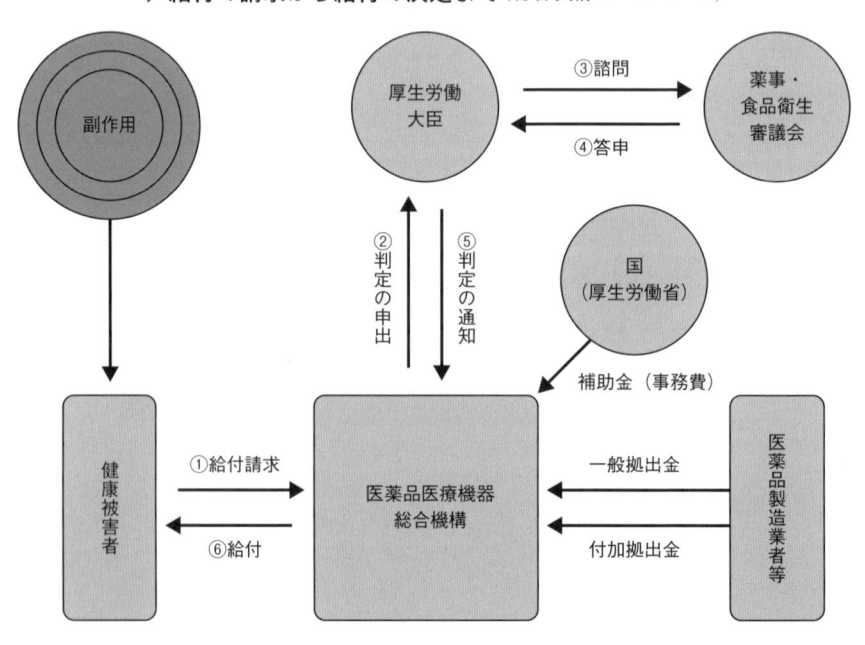

Summary of the Relief Service for Adverse Drug Reactions

The main requirements for payments are as follows:

(1) Cases where civil liability is difficult to prove, that is, cases where the MAHs or marketers of the drug concerned, medical institutions or other persons are clearly liable for damages are not eligible under this system.

(2) The use must have been "proper" (i. e. for an approved indication) . Cases where the product was used for an "improper purpose" (i. e. for an unapproved indication) or was used "improperly" in violation of the precautions for use of the drug are not eligible for this system.

(3) "ADRs, " harmful reactions caused by the pharmacological action of the drug, are covered, but "infections" due to contamination of the drug with bacteria or viruses or contamination due to foreign matter are not eligible for this system.

(4) Among ADRs, "damage requiring treatment equivalent to hospitalization," "disability of the first or second grade, that is, degree that markedly hinders activities of daily living or greater" and "death" are covered but mild ADRs are not eligible for this system.

(5) ADRs that are not "tolerable" are covered. ADRs that are considered appropriate to "tolerate" because they are a necessary part of treatment such as adverse reactions (ARs) due to drug (excluded drugs) such as anticancer drugs that must be used even though they have severe ARs and ADRs due to use of drugs in doses exceeding the usual dose in order to save the patient's life are not subject to this system. Anticancer drugs and immunosuppressants are among those designated as "excluded drugs."

A summary of the process is shown in **Fig**. It is necessary for an applicant to obtain a diagnostic report from

▶ **Process from application through decision on benefits** (PMDA web page)

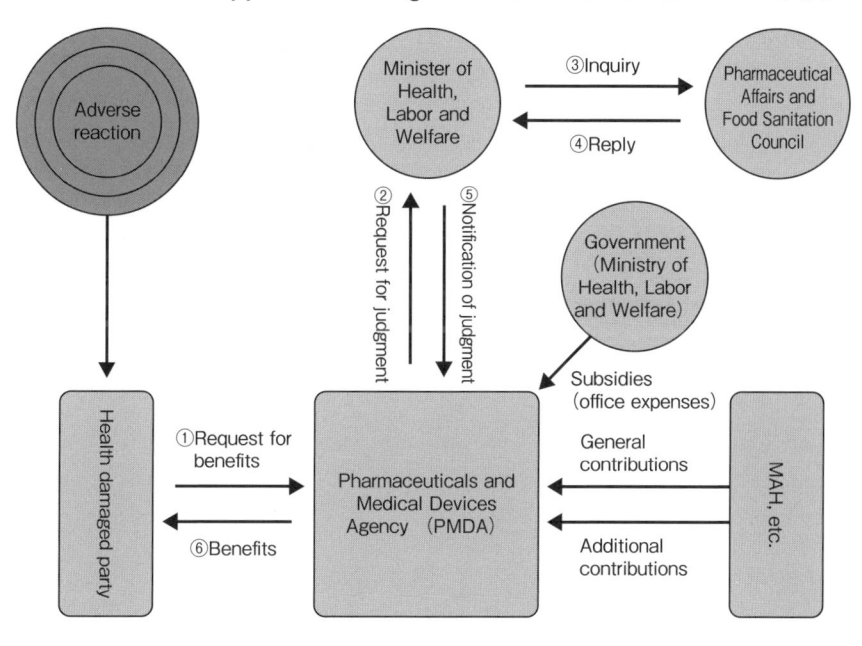

支給される給付には以下の種類がある.
①疾病(入院を必要とする程度)について医療を受けた場合—医療費,医療手当
②一定程度の障害(日常生活が著しく制限される程度以上のもの)の場合—障害年金,障害児養育年金
③死亡した場合—遺族年金,遺族一時金,葬祭料

医療費等の給付に必要な費用は,許可医薬品製造販売業者からの拠出金で賄われている.

次いで,2004年4月に新たに生物由来製品感染等被害救済制度が創設された.生物由来製品を適正に使用したにもかかわらず,その製品を介した感染により生じた,入院が必要な程度の疾病や障害などの健康被害について救済を行う制度である.また,感染後の発症を予防するための治療や二次感染者なども救済の対象となる.

本制度の財源は,許可生物由来製品製造販売業者からの拠出金で賄われている.

the physician who treated the AR, and a drug administration certificate. Therefore, he/she has to obtain cooperation from such physicians.

The following types of benefits are paid.
(1) Cases where treatment was received for a disease (severity requiring hospitalization)—Medical expenses, medical allowances
(2) Cases of disability to a certain degree (degree that markedly hinders activities of daily living or greater)—Disability pension, disabled child rearing pension
(3) Cases leading to death—Survivor pensions, survivor lump sum payments, funeral expenses

The funds necessary for paying benefits such as medical expenses are obtained from general contributions made by MAHs of licensed drugs.

And, then, a new Relief Service System for Infections derived from Biological Product was established in April 2004. This system provides relief for health damage such as diseases and disorders of sufficient severity to require hospitalization or the equivalent when infections occur via the product in spite of its proper use, and treatment to prevent onset after infection and patients with secondary infections. The finance resources of this system are general contributions made by MAHs of licensed biological products.

PMDAの理念

　わたしたちは，以下の行動理念のもと，医薬品，医療機器等の審査及び安全対策，並びに健康被害救済の三業務を公正に遂行し，国民の健康・安全の向上に積極的に貢献します。

・国民の命と健康を守るという絶対的な使命感に基づき，医療の進歩を目指して，判断の遅滞なく，高い透明性の下で業務を遂行します。
・より有効で，より安全な医薬品・医療機器をより早く医療現場に届けることにより，患者にとっての希望の架け橋となるよう努めます。
・最新の専門知識と叡智をもった人材を育みながら，その力を結集して，有効性，安全性について科学的視点で的確な判断を行います。
・国際調和を推進し，積極的に世界に向かって期待される役割を果たします。
・過去の多くの教訓を生かし，社会に信頼される事業運営を行います。

Our philosophy (PMDA)

PMDA continues to improve the public health and safety of our nation by reviewing applications for marketing approval of pharmaceuticals and medical devices, conducting safety measures, and providing relief to people who have suffered from adverse drug reactions.

We conduct our mission in accordance with the following principles:

- We pursue the development of medical science while performing our duty with greater transparency based on our mission to protect public health and the lives of our citizens.
- We will be the bridge between the patients and their wishes for faster access to safer and more effective drugs and medical devices.
- We make science-based judgments on quality, safety, and efficacy of medical products by training personnel to have the latest technical knowledge and wisdom in their field of expertise.
- We play an active role within the international community by promoting international harmonization.
- We conduct services in a way that is trusted by the public based on our experiences from the past.

▶ 日本の薬害年表

年	薬害関連の出来事	その他の出来事
1945		日本降伏, 連合国占領
46		
47		
48		旧薬事法制定
49		
1950		
51	ジフテリア予防接種禍事件	
52	｜	
53	｜ ペニシリンショック事件	
54	｜ ｜	
55	｜ ｜	
56	｜ ｜	水俣病
57	｜ ｜	
58	｜ ｜	
59	｜	
1960		現行薬事法制定
61		国民皆保険制度
62		
63		
64		ライシャワー大使刺傷事件
65	スモン事件 アンプル入り風邪薬事件 サリドマイド事件 クロロキンによる網膜障害	
66	｜ ｜ ｜ ｜	
67	｜ ｜ ｜ ｜ ストレプトマイシン聴力障害事件	
68	｜ ｜ ｜	カネミ油症事件
69	｜ ｜ ｜	
1970	｜ 種痘禍事件 ｜ ｜	四日市喘息／医薬品被害救済基金
71	｜ ｜ ｜	
72	｜ ｜ ｜ クロラムフェニコール再生不良貧血事件	
73	｜ ｜ ｜ ｜	
74	｜ 筋短縮症事件 ｜ ｜	
75	｜ ｜ DPTワクチン事故 ｜	
76	｜ ｜ ｜ ｜	
77	｜ ｜ ｜ ｜	

▶ Chronological Table of Drug-Induced Suffering in Japan

Year	Events related to drug-induced suffering							Other events
1945								Japan surrendered and was occupied by the Allied Powers
46								
47								
48								The old Pharmaceutical Affairs Law was established.
49	Diphtheria immunization incident							
1950								
51								
52								
53								
54			Penicillin shock incident					
55								
56								Minamata disease
57								
58								
59								
1960								The current Pharmaceutical Affairs Law was established.
61								Universal public insurance system was established.
62								
63								
64								Edwin O. Reischauer, American Ambassador to Japan, was assaulted and injured.
65		SMON incident	Cold-medicines-in-ampoules incident	Thalidomide incident	Retinal disorder caused by chloroquine			
66								
67						Streptomycin caused hearing loss incident		
68								Kanemi oil poisoning incident
69								
1970			Smallpox vaccination incident					Yokkaichi asthma
71								
72							Chloramphenicol caused aplastic anemia incident	The Fund for Relief Services for Adverse Drug Reactions
73								
74			Muscle contracture incident					
75				DPT vaccine accidents				
76								
77								

249

年	薬害関連の出来事							その他の出来事
78		スモン事件		DPTワクチン事故			クロラムフェニコール再生不良貧血	
79								
1980								
81								
82		ダイアライザー眼障害						
83								
84								
85								
86								
87								
88								
89								
1990				MMRワクチン事件	エイズ事件			
91								
92								
93		ソリブジン事件	陣痛促進剤事件					
94						イリノテカン骨髄抑制		
95								
96								
97	C型肝炎事件	トリグリタゾンによる肝障害					CJD事件	PMDA設置/審査業務開始
98								薬事法改正
99							ウシ心嚢膜による抗酸菌様感染	
2000								
1								産科医療補償制度
2								
3								
4								
5								
6		イレッサ事件						
7								
8								
9								
2010								
11								
12								
13								

chapter 4 • REFERENCE DATA

Year	Events related to drug-induced suffering							Other events
78		SMON incident		DPT vaccine accidents			Chloramphenicol caused aplastic anemia incident	
79		SMON incident		DPT vaccine accidents			Chloramphenicol caused aplastic anemia incident	
1980				DPT vaccine accidents			Chloramphenicol caused aplastic anemia incident	
81							Chloramphenicol caused aplastic anemia incident	
82		Dialyzer Induced Ophthalmologic Disorders Incident					Chloramphenicol caused aplastic anemia incident	
83							Chloramphenicol caused aplastic anemia incident	
84							Chloramphenicol caused aplastic anemia incident	
85							Chloramphenicol caused aplastic anemia incident	
86							Chloramphenicol caused aplastic anemia incident	
87							Chloramphenicol caused aplastic anemia incident	
88							Chloramphenicol caused aplastic anemia incident	
89							Chloramphenicol caused aplastic anemia incident	
1990				MMR vaccine incident	AIDS incident		Chloramphenicol caused aplastic anemia incident	
91				MMR vaccine incident	AIDS incident		Chloramphenicol caused aplastic anemia incident	
92				MMR vaccine incident	AIDS incident		Chloramphenicol caused aplastic anemia incident	
93	Blood product (fibrinogen) induced HCV infection incident	Sorivudine Incident	Labor-Inducing Drugs Incident		AIDS incident	Bone marrow suppression caused by irinotecan		
94	Blood product (fibrinogen) induced HCV infection incident		Labor-Inducing Drugs Incident		AIDS incident	Bone marrow suppression caused by irinotecan		
95	Blood product (fibrinogen) induced HCV infection incident		Labor-Inducing Drugs Incident		AIDS incident	Bone marrow suppression caused by irinotecan		
96	Blood product (fibrinogen) induced HCV infection incident		Labor-Inducing Drugs Incident			Bone marrow suppression caused by irinotecan	Human dried dura mater induced prion infection (CJD) incident	
97	Blood product (fibrinogen) induced HCV infection incident	Hepatic disorder caused by troglitazone	Labor-Inducing Drugs Incident			Bone marrow suppression caused by irinotecan	Human dried dura mater induced prion infection (CJD) incident	PMDA was established and started the reviews and related services.
98	Blood product (fibrinogen) induced HCV infection incident	Hepatic disorder caused by troglitazone	Labor-Inducing Drugs Incident			Bone marrow suppression caused by irinotecan		The Pharmaceutical Affairs Law was amended.
99	Blood product (fibrinogen) induced HCV infection incident	Hepatic disorder caused by troglitazone	Labor-Inducing Drugs Incident			Bone marrow suppression caused by irinotecan	Incident of bovine pericardium induced infection with probably acid-fast bacilli	
2000	Blood product (fibrinogen) induced HCV infection incident	Hepatic disorder caused by troglitazone	Labor-Inducing Drugs Incident			Bone marrow suppression caused by irinotecan	Incident of bovine pericardium induced infection with probably acid-fast bacilli	
1	Blood product (fibrinogen) induced HCV infection incident	Hepatic disorder caused by troglitazone	Labor-Inducing Drugs Incident			Bone marrow suppression caused by irinotecan	Incident of bovine pericardium induced infection with probably acid-fast bacilli	The Japan Obstetric Compensation System for Cerebral Palsy
2	Blood product (fibrinogen) induced HCV infection incident							
3	Blood product (fibrinogen) induced HCV infection incident							
4	Blood product (fibrinogen) induced HCV infection incident							
5	Blood product (fibrinogen) induced HCV infection incident	Iressa Incident						
6	Blood product (fibrinogen) induced HCV infection incident	Iressa Incident						
7	Blood product (fibrinogen) induced HCV infection incident	Iressa Incident						
8	Blood product (fibrinogen) induced HCV infection incident	Iressa Incident						
9	Blood product (fibrinogen) induced HCV infection incident	Iressa Incident						
2010		Iressa Incident						
11		Iressa Incident						
12		Iressa Incident						
13		Iressa Incident						

利益相反について

　本書を企画，執筆，出版した一般財団法人 医薬品医療機器レギュラトリーサイエンス財団の沿革と事業について以下の紹介を行うとともに，本書の発行に利益相反がないことを言明します。

財団の沿革

1956年　財団法人日本公定書協会として設立認可。東京に事務所設立。日本薬局方に関する情報提供，普及，啓発を目的とした活動を開始。
1991年　国立医薬品食品衛生研究所から日本薬局方の標準品製造，頒布の事業が部分的に移管される。大阪に分室を設けて事業開始。
1997年　JMO事業(ICH用国際医薬用語集の維持・管理・提供)を開始。
2004年　国立医薬品食品衛生研究所から標準品事業が全面的に移管される。
2006年　製薬企業の開発，品質管理，安全性担当者を対象とした薬事エキスパート研修会(現　レギュラトリーサイエンスエキスパート研修会)を開始。
2011年　一般財団法人に移行。名称を「医薬品医療機器レギュラトリーサイエンス財団」に変更。

PMRJ Declaration of Conflict of Interest

PMRJ Declaration of Conflict of Interest

The history and business of the Pharmaceutical and Medical Device Regulatory Science Society of Japan (PMRJ) that planned, authored, and published this book are introduced below. The PMRJ declares that there have been no conflicts of interest in the planning, writing or publication of this book.

History of the PMRJ

1956 The predecessor of the PMRJ, i.e. the Society of Japanese Pharmacopoeia (SJP), an incorporated foundation, was established and authorized. The SJP set up its office in Tokyo and started its activities for the purposes of providing information on the Japanese Pharmacopoeia (JP), making the JP widespread, and promoting public awareness of the JP.

1991 Part of the business of producing and distributing the Japanese Pharmacopoeia Reference Standards that was performed by the National Institute of Health Sciences was transferred to the SJP, which then established its Osaka Annex Office to start the transferred business.

1997 The Japanese Maintenance Organization (JMO) was established in the SJP and started the JMO business (i.e. maintenance, management, and provision of MedDRA/J (Japanese version of the Medical Dictionary for Regulatory Activities developed by the International Conference on Harmonization (ICH)).

2004 The whole business regarding the Japanese Pharmacopoeia Reference Standards was transferred from the National Institute of Health Sciences to the SJP.

2006 The SJP began to hold Educational Symposiums for Experts in Pharmaceutical Affairs (currently named "Educational Symposiums for Experts in Regulatory Science") which are designed for individuals engaged in development, quality control, and safety in pharmaceutical companies.

2011 The SJP was changed from an incorporated foundation to a general incorporated foundation in line with the legal change, and changed its name to the "Pharmaceutical and Medical Device Regulatory Science Society of Japan (PMRJ)".

財団の主な事業

1. **研修・認定事業**
   - レギュラトリーサイエンスエキスパート研修会(専門コース,特別コース)の開催
   - 日本薬局方に関する説明会,ICH即時報告会等の開催
   - 技術研修会の開催
   - レギュラトリーサイエンスエキスパート(開発,品質,PV)認定事業

2. **標準品事業**
   - 日本薬局方標準品等の製造・頒布
   - 標準品及びその取扱いに関する技術情報の発信
   - 外国薬局方標準品及び不純物標準品の取次販売

3. **刊行物発刊及び出版事業**
   - 月刊機関紙「医薬品医療機器レギュラトリーサイエンス」の発刊
   - 「日本薬局方フォーラム」の発刊
   - その他不定期の出版(日英対訳日本における医薬品リスクマネジメント等)

4. **調査研究事業**
   - 日本薬局方の試験法等の改正
   - レギュラトリーサイエンスの普及と推進のための調査研究

5. **JMO事業**
   - ICH国際医薬用語集(MedDRA/J)の提供及び維持管理

Major Business Activities of the PMRJ

1. Training & Certification Business Activity

- Holding Educational Symposiums for Experts in Regulatory Science (specific topic course and special course)
- Holding explanatory meetings on the Japanese Pharmacopoeia, briefing sessions immediately after ICH meetings, etc.
- Holding technical training sessions, etc.
- Issuing certificate of Regulatory Science Expert (in Clinical Development, Quality, and Pharmacovigilance (PV) fields)

2. Reference Standards Business Activity

- Production and distribution of the Japanese Pharmacopoeia Reference Standards, etc.
- Dissemination of technical information on the Reference Standards and how to handle them
- Acting as a distributor for the reference standards of overseas pharmacopoeias and the impurity reference materials

3. Publication Business Activity

- Publication of a monthly journal entitled "Pharmaceutical and Medical Device Regulatory Science"
- Publication of the "Japanese Pharmacopoeial Forum"
- Other publications issued irregularly ("Drug Risk Management in Japan (with English translation)", etc.)

4. Investigation & Research Business Activity

- Investigation and research relating to revision of testing methods, etc. of the Japanese Pharmacopoeia
- Investigation and research for the purpose of promoting regulatory science

5. JMO Business Activity

- Provision, maintenance, and management of MedDRA/J (Japanese version of the Medical Dictionary for Regulatory Activities developed by the International Conference on Harmonization (ICH))

執筆者略歴 (姓のアルファベット順)

Short curriculum vitae of Authors (in alphabetical order)

土井　脩　一般財団法人　医薬品医療機器レギュラトリーサイエンス財団　理事長

　1969年東京大学大学院薬学系研究科修士課程修了。薬学博士。東京大学応用微生物研究所において緑膿菌の抗生物質耐性機構を解明。その後，国立予防衛生研究所，ワシントン大学医学部を経て，1979年，審査官として厚生省本省勤務。1990年より審査第一課長・新医薬品課長としてICHを推進。安全課長，麻薬課長，大臣官房審議官(薬務担当，医薬安全担当)，医薬品医療機器総合機構理事(技監)，日本公定書協会専務理事を経て，2007年より現職。

Osamu Doi, Ph.D

Chief Executive
Pharmaceutical and Medical Device Regulatory Science Society of Japan (PMRJ)

Dr. Osamu Doi graduated from the Faculty of Pharmaceutical Sciences, University of Tokyo in 1967, and carried out research at the University's Institute of Applied Microbiology.　He was granted the Ph.D degree by the University of Tokyo.

Dr. Doi joined the National Institute of Health Japan as a researcher in 1969 and he has studied as a Postdoctoral Fellow at Washington University, St.Louis, USA.

Dr. Doi is Chief Executive of Pharmaceutical and Medical Device Regulatory Science Society of Japan (PMRJ)

Before this he was Chief Executive of the Society of Japanese Pharmacopoeia(SJP), Senior Executive Director of the SJP, Senior Executive Director of the Pharmaceuticals and Medical Devices Agency(PMDA), the Executive Director of the Organization for Pharmaceutical Safety and Research(OPSR), Councilor for Pharmaceutical and Medical Safety of the Ministry of Health and Welfare, Councilor for Pharmaceutical Affairs of the same Ministry, Councilor of the Organization for ADR Relief, R & D Promotion and Product Review, Director of the Narcotics Division, Safety Division, New Drugs Division, First Evaluation and Registration Division of the Pharmaceutical Affairs Bureau, and Director of the Office of Environmental Chemicals Safety in the Environmental Health Bureau of the Ministry of Health and Welfare.

木村　暁　一般財団法人　医薬品医療機器レギュラトリーサイエンス財団　参事

　1972年大阪大学基礎工学部生物工学科卒業。2013年大阪大学大学院人間科学研究科博士前期課程修了。ダイナボット，アストラ，アストラゼネカにて学術，臨床開発，安全性情報(治験薬，市販薬)業務に従事。その後ベルメディカルソリューションを経て，2011年より現職。

Satoru Kimura

Counselor

Pharmaceutical and Medical Device Regulatory Science Society of Japan (PMRJ)

Mr. Kimura graduated from the Division of Biophysical Engineering, School of Engineering Science, Osaka University in 1972. He completed the first half period of his Doctor's Program in human science at the Graduate School of Human Science of Osaka University in 2013.

Mr. Kimura was engaged in duties related to scientific affairs, clinical development, and safety information (investigational and marketed products) at Dainabot, Astra, and AstraZeneca.

Mr. Kimura has been Counselor of the Pharmaceutical and Medical Device Regulatory Science Society of Japan (PMRJ) since 2011. Before this post, he worked at Bell Medical Solutions.

小山　弘子　一般財団法人　医薬品医療機器レギュラトリーサイエンス財団
　　　　　　参事兼研修企画コーディネーター

　1967年千葉大学薬学部薬学科卒業。杏林化学で研究所勤務(毒性・薬物代謝，研究企画に従事)。1970年同社を退職後，日本ロシュに入社。1994年まで医薬品本部に在籍し，1979年まで学術関連業務。1980年から市販後調査業務に従事。1995～2002年10月の中外製薬との合併まで，開発本部で治験薬・市販薬の安全性業務に従事。2008年3月まで中外製薬信頼性保証本部等にてグローバルファーマコビジランスを担当。またファーマコビジランス関係のICH-topicsに日本製薬工業会の代表として参加。2008年より現職。

Hiroko Koyama, RPh

Counselor

Training & Planning Coordinator

Pharmaceutical and Medical Device Regulatory Science Society of Japan (PMRJ)

Ms. Koyama graduated from the Faculty of Pharmaceutical Sciences, Chiba University in 1967, registered pharmacist since 1968.

Ms. Koyama joined Kyorin Chemical Laboratories as a researcher in 1967 and spent 3 years. She joined Nippon Roche in 1970 and retired from Chugai (Roche Group from 2002) in 2008. She was vice-chairperson of PMS sub-committee, Drug Evaluation Committee, JPMA , topic leader of ICH-E2B (M) IWG, deputy topic leader of ICH-E2B (R) EWG from JPMA and ICH-Risk Communication

IWG rapporteur.

Ms. Koyama is counselor, training and planning coordinator of the Pharmaceutical and Medical Device Regulatory Science Society of Japan (PMRJ).

Before this post, she was Senior Leader of Drug Safety Unit of Chugai Pharmaceutical Co., Ltd. (Chugai), Senior Leader of Drug Safety Evaluation Department of Chugai, Head of Drug Safety Department of Nippon Roche(Roche Japan), General Manager of Post-marketing Surveillance (Roche Japan), Product Manager of Benzodiazepines(Roche Japan), and Head of Medical Information Service Section (Roche Japan).

She was a member of science research project on Package Insert, Patient Package Insert and Drug-Drug Interactions sponsored by Ministry of Health and Welfare (MHW), and a member of science research project on Early Post-marketing Phase Vigilance sponsored by Ministry of Health, Labor and Welfare (MHLW). She was a core-committee member of Clinical Safety and Pharmacovigilance SIAC of DIA, and a member of program committee of DIA Japan Annual Meeting.

最上　紀美子　一般財団法人　医薬品医療機器レギュラトリーサイエンス財団
　　　　　　　理事兼研修事業本部長

　1977年東京大学薬学部薬学科卒業。医学博士。1977年から1980年まで日本ロシュにて，研究所，医薬品本部に在籍し，学術関連業務に従事。1994～2004年まで山口大学医学部生理学第一講座(現：器官制御医科学講座生体機能分子制御学)にて助手，学内講師として研究および教育に従事。2006～2009年まで医薬品医療機器総合機構安全部医薬品安全課勤務。2009年日本公定書協会に勤務。2012年より現職。

Kimiko Mogami, Ph.D

Executive Director

Pharmaceutical and Medical Device Regulatory Science Society of Japan (PMRJ)

Dr. Mogami graduated from the Faculty of Pharmaceutical Sciences, University of Tokyo in 1977, registered pharmacist since 1977. She was granted the Ph.D degree by Yamaguchi University in 2002.

Dr. Mogami joined Nippon Roche in 1977 and spent 3 years and 9 months in Medical Information Service Section of Drug Safety Department. She joined Yamaguchi University of Medicine as Research Associate in 1994 and Assistant Professor in 2002 of 1st Department of Physiology (Molecular Physiology and Medical Bioregulation), and spent 10 and a half years.

Dr. Mogami is Executive Director of Pharmaceutical and Medical Device Regulatory Science Society of Japan (PMRJ).

Before this she was Director of Educational Activities for Pharmaceutical Professionals of PMRJ,

Director of the Society of Japanese Pharmacopoeia (SJP), Deputy Manager of SJP, and a stuff of Drug Safety Division of the Pharmaceuticals and Medical Devices Agency (PMDA).

野口　隆志　一般財団法人　医薬品医療機器レギュラトリーサイエンス財団
　　　　　　参事兼研修企画コーディネーター，昭和大学薬学部客員教授

　1965年京都薬科大学薬学部卒業。住友化学工業入社後，医薬事業部勤務。1984年分離合併により新設された住友製薬（現：大日本住友製薬）へ移籍。研究開発本部にて臨床開発業務に従事。医薬品開発，品質保証部，海外事業等の担当理事（本社支配人）を経て2003年定年退職。同年昭和大学薬学部客員教授（臨床薬学教室）（現在に至る）。同年11月，国際医療福祉大学大学院臨床試験研究分野（現：創薬育薬医療分野）教授及び薬学部教授を経て2009年定年退職。2009年より現職。

Takashi Noguchi
　Counselor
　Training & Planning Coordinator
　Pharmaceutical and Medical Device Regulatory Science Society of Japan (PMRJ)
　Visiting Professor at the School of Pharmaceutical Sciences, Showa University

Mr. Noguchi graduated from the Department of Pharmaceutical Sciences, Kyoto Pharmaceutical University in 1965.

Mr. Noguchi joined Sumitomo Chemical and worked at the Business Division of Drugs throughout his career at this company. In 1984, he was transferred to Sumitomo Pharmaceutical (presently: Dainippon Sumitomo Pharma) which was newly established due to merger of the companies. He was engaged in clinical development related duties at the Headquarters of Research and Development, and became the Director (General Manager at the Head Office) responsible for drug development, quality assurance, and overseas business activities. In 2003, he left the company since he reached the determined age of retirement.

Mr. Noguchi became Visiting Professor at the School of Pharmaceutical Sciences, Showa University (in the Section of Clinical Pharmaceutical Sciences) in 2003, which he continues to hold.

Mr. Noguchi is Counselor and Training & Planning Coordinator of the Pharmaceutical and Medical Device Regulatory science Society of Japan (PMRJ).

Before this Mr. Noguchi became Professor at Graduate School, International University of Health and Welfare (in the Field of Clinical Study Research which is presently the Field of Drug Discovery & Medical Care) in November 2003, and became Professor of the Faculty of Pharmaceutical Sciences. In 2009, he left the university since he reached the determined age of retirement.

津田　重城　一般財団法人　医薬品医療機器レギュラトリーサイエンス財団　専務理事

　1983年北海道大学大学院薬学研究科修士課程修了。同年厚生省入省後，安全課，大臣官房国際課，監視指導課等に勤務。1989～1992年OECD派遣。2004年医薬品医療機器総合機構品質管理部，企画調整部。2007年日本公定書協会で学術・研修部長などを経て，2012年より現職。

Shigeki Tsuda, M.S.

Senior Managing Director
Pharmaceutical and Medical Device Regulatory Science Society of Japan (PMRJ)

Mr. Tsuda graduated from the Faculty of Pharmaceutical Sciences, Hokkaido University in 1981 and received his Master degree of pharmaceutical sciences from the Graduate School of the same university in 1983.

Mr. Tsuda joined the (then) Ministry of Health and Welfare and spent 3 and a half years in Chemicals division, OECD (Organisation for Economic Co-operation and Development) in Paris, France.

Mr. Tsuda is Senior Managing Director of the Pharmaceutical and Medical Device Regulatory Science Society of Japan (PMRJ).

Before this post, he was Senior Executive Director of PMRJ and the Society of Japanese Pharmacopoeia (SJP), Director of Educational and Scientific Activities of the SJP, Director of International Affairs/ Human Resources Development Division of the Pharmaceuticals and Medical Devices Agency (PMDA), Director of Standards Division of PMDA, Deputy Director of the Office of Chemical Safety, Deputy Director of Safety Division and Deputy Director of Inspection and Guidance Division in the Pharmaceutical Safety Bureau, Deputy Director of International Affairs Division in Minister's Secretariat, and Assistant Director of Medical Economics Division in the Health Insurance Bureau.

翻　訳

北川　千里　　神戸市外国語大学外国語学部英米学科卒業。フリーランス翻訳者・通訳者。
　　　　　　　一般財団法人 日本翻訳連盟会員。

>Brief personal history of translator
>
>**Chisato Kitagawa**　　Graduated from the Department of English Studies, Kobe City University of Foreign Studies. Freelance technical interpreter/translator. Membership at the Japan Translation Federation (JTF), a general incorporated association.

編集担当

秋山　典子　　一般財団法人　医薬品医療機器レギュラトリーサイエンス財団　出版部長
　　　　　　　東邦大学薬学部薬学科卒業。薬剤師。

>Brief personal history of editor
>
>**Noriko Akiyama**　　Graduated from the Faculty of Pharmaceutical Sciences, Toho University. Pharmacist. Director of the Publication Division, Pharmaceutical and Medical Device Regulatory Science Society of Japan (PMRJ), a general incorporated foundation

日本の薬害事件
─薬事規制と社会的要因からの考察─

定価　本体10,000円（税別）

平成25年9月20日　第1版発行

企画・編集　一般財団法人 医薬品医療機器レギュラトリーサイエンス財団
　〒150-0002　東京都渋谷区渋谷2-12-15 日本薬学会 長井記念館
　電話 03-3400-5634　　URL　http://www.pmrj.jp

発　　行　株式会社 薬事日報社
　〒101-8648　東京都千代田区神田和泉町1番地
　電話 03-3862-2141　　URL　http://www.yakuji.co.jp

©2013　　　　　　　　　組版：㈱ビーコム　印刷：㈱日本制作センター
Printed in Japan

落丁・乱丁の場合は，お取り換えいたします．

Drug-Induced Suffering in Japan
─ A Review from Regulatory and Social Perspectives ─

ISBN 978-4-8408-1249-8　C3047

Copyright © 2013 by Pharmaceutical and Medical Device Regulatory Science Society of Japan

Edited by　Pharmaceutical and Medical Device Regulatory Science Society
　　　　　　of Japan (PMRJ)
　　　　　　2-12-15, Shibuya, Shibuya-ku, Tokyo 150-0002, Japan
　　　　　　TEL：＋81 3 3400 5634；FAX：＋81 3 3400 3158

Published by　YAKUJI NIPPO, LTD.
　　　　　　　1, Kanda Izumicho, Chiyoda-ku, Tokyo 101-8648, Japan